AVENGER

So far, his psychic powers have claimed twenty human killing monsters. As vicious as they were, they were no more than the agents of death. Today, he must face death himself. . . .

SURVIVOR

The key to the ultimate terror that stalks the city, she is the only woman who can redeem the heart of a redeemer.

TRACKER

For years he's relentlessly pursued the killer of serial killers. When tracker and target meet at last, they must become allies, and join forces—at least long enough to bring down the greatest evil of all.

➜ ➜ ➜

"Taut and mysterious. . . . It expertly keeps the reader in suspense."
—*Library Journal*

"Gripping and hard to put down."
—*StarPhoenix* (Canada)

"This book has a special aura about it...and would grace most any kind of 'Best 10' list anyone might compile."
—**Broox Sledge, "The Book World,"**
Neshoba Democrat-Philadelphia (MS)

PREDATORS

DAINA GRAZIUNAS
and JIM STARLIN

Originally published as *Thinning the Predators*

WARNER BOOKS

A Time Warner Company

The events and characters in this book are fictitious. Certain real locations and public figures are mentioned, but all other characters and the events described in the book are totally imaginary.

If you purchase this book without a cover you should be aware that this book may have been stolen property and reported as "unsold and destroyed" to the publisher. In such case neither the author nor the publisher has received any payment for this "stripped book."

WARNER BOOKS EDITION

Cover design and illustration by Tony Greco

Warner Books, Inc.
1271 Avenue of the Americas
New York, NY 10020

Visit our Web site at
http://pathifinder.com/twep

W A Time Warner Company

Printed in the United States of America

Originally published in hardcover under the title, *Thinning the Predators*, by Warner Books.
First Paperback Printing: July, 1997

10 9 8 7 6 5 4 3 2 1

*To all our friends, especially
Mary Jo Duffy, Dottye Howard, and Ron Marz,
for all their help and encouragement*

PREDATORS

PART ONE

Metempsychosis

*In our sad condition our only consolation
is the expectancy of another life.*

—Martin Luther

PART ONE

Metempsychosis

1

JUNE 23, 1996
JUST OUTSIDE INDIAN SPRINGS, NEVADA

Ira Levitt awoke in the near dark to a nasty surprise. His six-foot-five-inch frame was lying on the damp ground, his head throbbed, and his left arm felt broken. A fact confirmed when he tried to wriggle his fingers. Damn this work! They could just take this job and shove it. They who? Nobody was listening.

An almost full moon clearly illuminated his predicament. But the kettledrums in his head kept pounding as Ira lay there, remembering. First, the man stepping from behind the corner of the house, then the quick flash of a two-by-four as it swung wildly toward his head. The last thing Ira remembered was raising his arm instinctively to ward off the blow. The memory ended there.

Ira awkwardly hoisted his bulk into a sitting position and unbuttoned his shirt enough to gingerly slip his damaged arm inside. "Not tonight, Josephine," he muttered. "You see, I have this splitting headache." The thought caught him by surprise and almost made him giggle. But the fact that the man with the two-by-four might still be lurking nearby stilled it in his throat. Unfortunately, a rousing chorus of the "Marseillaise" was now playing in his brain. "Must be punch-drunk. That's it. Gotta get up and out of here. I'm getting too old for this shit, anyway."

So Ira Levitt, G-man with twenty-eight years' field experience at the Bureau, stood up feeling wobbly, minus his flashlight and gun, and cautiously picked his way back to where he had left Officers Bacon and Goddin of the Indian Springs PD. They had brought him out here a mere half hour ago, according to his digital watch. A Timex. Takes a lickin' and keeps on tickin'. Ira hoped Bacon and Goddin were that resilient. He wondered if they were still alive.

Alive, yes. Happy, no. Both men sat propped up against a tree, bare-chested. Their uniform shirts had been pressed into emergency service as bandages and were wrapped around their right thighs. The moonlight glinted off two service revolvers. "Take it easy, men," Ira said as he approached. "It's me. Levitt."

"Levitt! And just where the hell have you been, huh?"

Ira couldn't remember if this irate law enforcement officer was Bacon or Goddin. He'd met them just this afternoon, and right now his head wasn't working at peak efficiency. There was quite a bit of ringing going on in there, and an occasional "*Allons, enfants de la patrie . . .*"

"Got beaned with a piece of lumber," Ira answered wearily. He had a terrible feeling this whole mess was going to end up being blamed on him. "What happened here?"

"Bacon and I were waiting for you to return, exactly where you left us. We heard the shot. So we came to back you up. Got this far when we heard someone approaching. We took cover. The guy coming from the house, whoever he was, called out our names. Sounded like he was in pain. Figured it had to be you, so we stepped out of the bushes, and whammo . . . we find ourselves blinded by the glare of a flashlight. Next thing we know, we've each got a bullet in the leg for our trouble."

Ira bent over to look at Officer Goddin's wound in the pale moonlight. All he said was "So he knew your names, eh?"

Goddin didn't even try to conceal the instantaneous dislike for Ira that the big man had sensed when they'd first met. "Yeah, how you suppose he knew that? You holding out on us?" Locals versus the Feds. Old interagency hatreds and suspicions never fade.

"Easy, boys, I'm on your side," Ira said with a rueful smile. "So I'm going to let the last question pass unanswered and uncommented upon. 'Cause let's face it, we're none of us in any condition to step out into the alley and settle this like men. Okay? Oh, and Goddin . . . don't ever let anyone tell you that you're not a *mensch*."

Levitt, uncharacteristically stoop-shouldered, feeling both his age and his little joust with Goddin, shuffled over to Officer Bacon and cursorily examined the second man's leg wound. Pretty fancy shooting, this. We're talking marksmanship medal. Each man's bullet had struck the outer edge of the right thigh, incapacitating its quarry with a minimum of injury. Nicely done. Clean, thorough, effective, yet almost polite. From the bloodstains soaking the shirts, Ira could tell that each leg had both an entrance and an exit wound. The bullets had passed through without stopping. Thank God for small favors. At least ballistics wouldn't be able to prove definitively that it was his gun that had downed these men. In the long run, though, that didn't really matter. Ira knew the truth and would have to live with it. He looked into Officer Bacon's angry eyes and said, "I guess you've already called in for backup?"

Bacon glared at Levitt. "I'd like to know how you expect us to do that. The creep that popped us took off in the cruiser!"

"He what?" Ira was finding it hard to keep a straight face. The cheeky bastard had done it again.

"Stole the damn patrol car! You deaf or something? After he plugged us, he circled around to the car. We took a few wild shots at him in the dark, but we didn't have a chance in hell of hitting him. A moment or so later we heard the engine start up and the car drive off. We've been sitting here ever since, wondering what the fuck we should do."

Ira got to his feet and looked in the direction he'd come from. "I'll head back to the house and call for help. Let me borrow a gun and a flashlight."

Officer Goddin sullenly produced the two desired items without comment. Ira accepted them in the spirit in which they were offered and turned to go. But he took only a few steps before he turned and over his shoulder said, "When the shooter was going through the brush, how did he sound?"

"Oh . . . yeah! That's right!"

Ira was too far away to see Officer Bacon's face light up, but he could hear the recognition in the man's voice. "He was limping," Bacon said. "Or maybe dragging one leg. Say, did you tag him?"

"I'm not sure. Look, sit tight. I'll be back for you in a few."

❧❧❧❧

Ira made his way back to the Keefer house, flashlight in hand, Goddin's gun stuffed inside his belt. A trace of a smile played around the edges of his mouth. He had a dim recollection of his gun discharging just as that two-by-four crashed into his arm and head.

When he reached the darkened farmhouse, Ira returned to the corner where he'd been waylaid. A quick flick of the flashlight simply confirmed what he already knew down deep in his kishkes: his own pistol and flashlight were gone. Dammit! What a mess!

Kishkes. They serve you well in this line of work. Yiddish word. Means guts. Guts, gut instinct, intestinal fortitude, intuition, all that good stuff. Hell of a lot more accurate, too, than some "little voice." Kishkes never lie.

The borrowed flashlight also revealed something that lightened Ira's mood considerably: blood. It stained the grass and it didn't belong to him. Since Bacon and Goddin hadn't made it this far, that left only one possibility. His reflexive shot had found its mark. Ira had managed to tag the man he'd traveled all the way from Washington, D.C., to bust. His quarry had escaped, but not completely unscathed. Ira, though not yet successful in his relentless pursuit of David Vandemark, had at least left his prey, this time, with a little something to remember him by. Cold comfort, perhaps, but sometimes you've got to take what you can get.

Ira flicked off the flashlight, jammed it awkwardly into his pants pocket, and pulled the gun from his belt. He didn't really think he'd need it, but he wasn't one of those John Wayne types who took unnecessary chances. As far as

Ira was concerned, being macho was the surest way to get cheated out of your pension. Besides, enough had already gone wrong tonight. Entering this house without a drawn gun would be plain foolish. After all, this was the home of a mass murderer. A serial killer. Why else would David Vandemark have come here?

∽∾∾∽

Levitt found the front door open and quietly stepped inside, into the foyer's deepest shadows. He stood there, stock-still, listening.

Only one faint repetitive sound reached his straining ears—dripping: *dap, dap, dap, dap, dap.*

Aside from that, the house was as quiet as a tomb. Ira immediately regretted this careless thought. It heightened his already excruciating feeling of claustrophobia. Gun at the ready, he silently inched his way down the hallway, coming steadily closer to the sound of the dripping. *Dap, dap, dap.*

Ira peered into the room at the end of the hall. The moonlight drifting in through the windows revealed that this was the kitchen, but he couldn't make out any details. The faint light of an illuminated switch cast an eerie glow on the far wall, near the back door. The dripping sound was much more distinct now. Ira knew it was probably just a worn washer in the kitchen sink. Still, the sound grated unbearably on his taut nerves. *Dap, dap, dap.* Funny, it didn't sound much like water dripping on porcelain.

He glided across the room, surprisingly light-footed for a man his size. Ira's eyes noted the dull white of the kitchen sink to his right. He stood there for a moment, once again listening for sounds of movement elsewhere in the house. Nothing but the sound of the dripping reached him. *Dap, dap, dap.*

It registered suddenly that the annoying drip wasn't coming from the sink. It was coming from the darkened corner at the far side of the room. Ira's eyes tried to penetrate that gloom. The effort made his head throb. He finally conceded that the only way to find out what was making that noise was to turn on either the kitchen light or his flashlight. With only one good arm, using the latter would mean putting down the gun, a flawed idea at best. The switch for the kitchen light, however, was only inches to the left of where Ira was standing.

Dap, dap, dap.

Ira squeezed his eyes shut, bent his knees, letting his back touch the wall, and slid along it to his left until the light switch poked him in the shoulder blade. As he straightened up, he felt the switch flip upward. Let there be light. And so there was, on the other side of his closed eyelids. When he opened his eyes, Ira blinked at the glare, and then at the awful truth.

Dap, dap, dap, dap, dap.

Blood dripped freely from the kitchen table onto the sheet of black plastic that covered the floor. The savagery of the scene made Ira stare, dumbly uncomprehending for several seconds, and then gag as the full impact of it hit him. Ira felt his stomach revolt, seeking an easy out. He looked away and pressed the back of his hand to his mouth. Hold it down. Not in here. God, he hated this, coming onto the scene of a fresh murder. This was one of those times when he had to ask himself why. Why had he

chosen this *farchadat* line of work? Oh, God, this one had
to be the worst he'd ever seen.

Ira slowly turned his head back toward the grisly sight
of the naked teenage boy lying across the table, staring
blindly up at the ceiling. At least what was left of the boy
lay on the table.

Dap, dap, dap, dap, dap.

The steady dripping combined with Ira's own heartbeat,
which was thudding in his ears for a jolly rendition of the
Anvil Chorus. He rubbed his gun hand against his head, to
make it go away. The flat, cool metal of the pistol felt good
against his right temple. The room was close, so close, and
everywhere that smell. The teenager's limbs had been
crudely sawed off. Two large stainless-steel buckets sat on
the floor. One was carelessly jammed full of bloody bones
with bits of muscle tissue still hanging from them. The
other was nearly full of what appeared to be chopped meat.

Ira stared at the grim tableau, still not fully compre-
hending. But then he noticed the industrial-size meat
grinder bolted to the kitchen table. Its gruesome presence
tore away all of Ira's emotional blinders with a single rip.
Like removing a Band-Aid. "My God . . . my God . . ."

The FBI agent felt himself sway, suddenly dizzy, and
steadied himself against what he presumed was the refrigerator. But the refrigerator was on the other side of the room.
Then what the hell was this? Ira turned and saw that he was
leaning against a stand-up freezer, the kind in which sane
folks kept a king's ransom in steaks and other prime cuts.

He opened the freezer door with a solemn deliberate-
ness and looked in at the neatly wrapped packages. Then
with the same quiet dignity he closed the door. "You
stinking crazy bastard. All those young lives . . ." Ira

glanced over again at the poor butchered boy. One huge tear he'd been struggling against so fiercely rolled sadly, silently down his cheek and onto his chin.

As Ira wiped it away, he glanced down at the floor and saw bloody footprints leading away from the kitchen table. "You son of a bitch," he said quietly, "I hope you're still here," and he followed the tracks out of the kitchen.

They led into the living room, where Ira found a man sitting on the floor, his back against one side of the mantelpiece. A shotgun was lying across his lap, and there was a small bullet hole in the middle of his forehead. A tiny trickle of blood had crawled down the man's face, mingling with the boy's blood, which stained his white shirt and butcher's apron. Over the fireplace hung an empty gun rack. David Vandemark had given his latest quarry more than a sporting chance at freedom before killing him. This fairness had become David's trademark, almost a signature. Ira looked over his shoulder and saw where the shotgun blast had peppered the wall. He was once again left to ponder something he'd wondered about countless times before: was David Vandemark, the blade-running vigilante, playing Russian roulette with a heavy death wish, or was his overly keen sense of fair play a way of gaining some kind of ritualistic psychosexual thrill that heightened the pleasure of his vengeance?

Ira looked down at the corpse without regret and without pity. This would be Elmore Keefer, the house's owner. It was Keefer's clandestine activities that had drawn both David Vandemark and Ira Levitt to this lonely section of Nevada tonight. Teenagers, boys and girls both, had been disappearing around these parts for the last eighteen months. State police had come to the conclusion that these kids had probably vanished while hitchhiking along the interstate. But Ira knew that if the disappearances were in fact the work of a serial killer, Vandemark would be unable to resist the mystery.

So Levitt, following this hunch, had arrived a week ago in Indian Springs in the hope of setting a trap. Earlier in the day he'd happened upon a gas station attendant who remembered that someone vaguely matching Vandemark's description had asked about an Elmore Keefer. That tip had led Ira to this farmhouse. One step behind Vandemark.

Ira Levitt, warm, compassionate, feeling human being, was glad things had worked out the way they had. While Ira Levitt, federal law enforcement officer, sworn to uphold the letter of the law, was pissed off, seething with disappointment at having failed to bag his prey. Again.

He'd been tracking David Vandemark for the past seven years. He'd had a seven-year love-hate relationship with a man he'd never even seen face to face until tonight. Ira looked at his injured arm. "So what happens when we finally meet?" he groused. "I let him break my arm. What a schmuck!"

Ira found a phone in the bedroom and called for ambulances and backup. Then he wandered out onto the front porch and sat down on the steps to await the cavalry's arrival. The cool night breeze felt good after the stagnant stink of that slaughterhouse. Ira breathed deeply, filling his lungs with the clean evening air. The stench, though, still hung in his nostrils.

He'd been so close this time. It would be humiliating, going back to Washington empty-handed, having to report yet another failure on the Vandemark case. Ira wondered if possibly David Vandemark might just outlast him.

2

The woman's mind was an open book to Roger Cordell. That was the name he was using for now. To Roger, names were like cars. When one outlived its usefulness, it was time to get another. He sneaked a peek at her out of the corner of his eye. She was a cute redhead in her midthirties. Long legs and a nice ass. Her thoughts were extremely sexual. Roger smiled at their carnality. Like waving a red flag at a bull, he thought.

He was standing in line at the minimart's checkout counter. Red was over by the magazine rack, leafing through a copy of *Cosmo*. But every few seconds or so, he could feel her eyes drift up from the pages to rest on him. She was checking him out: five feet eleven, sandy blond hair, dark tan, nicely trimmed Vandyke, strong cheekbones. Good build. Not too much muscle, but what was there was taut and wiry. She wished she could see his eyes. Those damned mirrored sunglasses.

Roger turned his gaze directly toward the woman, with an index finger slid the glasses down his aquiline nose, and gave her the full effect of his steely blue eyes. He used them in his work quite regularly, knew the impact they had.

Her reaction was immediate: she blushed bright crimson and looked away, crammed the magazine clumsily back into the rack, and practically ran out of the store. Roger savored the fear he had instilled in her. Married ladies shouldn't hang around grocery stores thinking about picking up strange men. Good way to catch something deadly.

He slid the glasses back into place. The checkout girl had begun to ring up his groceries. No reason to startle the pretty little bleached-blond register puncher. She was doing a slow enough job of toting up his bill, bored into minimum-wage semiconsciousness. When she was finished, Roger paid for the food and drink, picked up the twin grocery bags, and exited into the warm, muggy Florida air.

If his female admirer had lingered, she could have added a limp to her inventory of Roger's vital statistics. Roger noticeably favored his left leg as he made his way across the steamy parking lot to the Nissan. The car's rental agreement was in the name of Gregory Parsons, another of the man's many casual identities. Roger waited outside the vehicle for several minutes, until the air conditioning had somewhat managed to cool the blistering hotbox that the blazing tropical sun had made of the automobile. He lit a cigarette and stared dreamily at the small pond next to the parking lot. There was a notice posted at its center, advising people not to feed the alligators. He grinned, just as he had every time he'd seen that sign. Florida. What a weird place.

❧

Ten minutes later he checked to make certain the car was locked before exiting the visitors' parking area at the

Snook Motel, his home for the last three weeks. Roger limped over to the door of 1A, the first-floor room facing the ocean. He was glad he'd come to Sanibel to convalesce. Couldn't think of a better place in the world to let a bullet wound heal.

In the privacy of his room, Roger pulled off his slacks, unwrapped the bandages surrounding his left thigh, and examined the damaged goods. The wound was closed, and the seeping hadn't resumed. A good sign. He'd been walking around quite a bit today, running errands, and was afraid the strain might have been more than the leg was ready for just yet.

After all, it had only been three weeks, and the bullet remained lodged inside his thigh. Roger relaxed, lit another cigarette, and for easily the thousandth time, thought about the likelihood that this damn slug might remain a part of him for the rest of his life. He knew he couldn't remove it himself, and venal, unscrupulous Dr. Lipston, Roger's personal physician for nearly five years, to whom doctor-patient confidentiality was a sacred trust that he was willing to protect for the right price, had finally managed to drink himself to death last spring. This left Roger practically without access to professional treatment for the variety of dicey injuries he incurred on the job. He really missed that old sot sometimes. It wasn't easy finding a physician with such a cavalier attitude toward injuries of an obviously felonious origin.

Roger had tried to locate one when he first came to Florida with this federal .38 caliber bullet burning in his leg. But his brief search had proved fruitless, and he'd had to settle for his own ministrations. The years had taught him a few things about do-it-yourself repairs.

His efforts had succeeded. With what he'd picked up at a drugstore, he'd managed to stop the bleeding without having the leg turn gangrenous and fall off. Plenty of other people lived with bullets or shrapnel lodged in their bodies, bits of metal that couldn't be removed for various reasons. Roger was getting pretty comfortable with the idea; being an oddity was nothing new to him.

After rebandaging the leg, Roger slipped into a pair of cutoff dungarees, grabbed a cold can of Coors, and went down to the beach to work on his tan. He had baked himself to a deep bronze over the past few weeks, but he wanted to get even darker. He was already planning his next job, and this time it looked as if he'd have to pass for Hispanic in order to pull it off.

∞∞∞

A fat lady and a young couple with a little boy were already enjoying the sun and surf when Roger limped out onto the sandy stretch of beach. As he eased himself onto the lounge chair and took his first sip of beer, feeling deliciously lazy, he thought about how easy it would be to spend the rest of his life right here. To spend his time doing nothing but enjoying the sun and the beaches along the Gulf Coast. But that wasn't the way it was meant to be. Roger knew this.

A small muscle in his jaw danced as reality intruded on his wonderful daydream. He had a special calling. A God-given talent. The easy life wasn't in the cards for him. He'd accepted this fact years ago and had made accommodations for the myriad little and not-so-little problems it created. Sometimes Roger marveled at his own adaptability. He'd come a long way since those early days back in Warren, Michigan.

Roger watched a woman walk by on the beach. She was golden brown, leggy, very blond, and lost in thoughts of a hazel-eyed man she'd met earlier in the week. She slowly walked out of sight, out of mind.

Attitude—that was the key to success, according to Roger. It was attitude that had gotten him this far. The trick was to not take life all that seriously. Life arbitrarily gave you only what it felt like giving, he thought, so why waste a lot of time worrying about it? Roger liked to keep his mind on the job. Work was one thing over which he could retain some measure of control—much more than over any other aspect of his life. The only way to get through existence, then, was to enjoy the good parts and laugh at the bad ones and hope they'd soon pass. Savor living, but don't get too attached to any part of it. Because everything is so ephemeral.

David Vandemark couldn't accept this. Pain and loss had crushed the man. That was why David was dead. And why Roger now inhabited his body. Poor bastard, thought Roger. He couldn't live with the knowledge that life was a bad joke and the laugh was on him.

Roger stared at the blue-on-blue horizon, a smug grin on his face. Yes, the only way to get by was to learn to appreciate life's black humor.

Mrs. Emma Adler, an overweight widow from Newark, turned around in her beach chair and glowered at Roger. She suspected the drunken fool was laughing at her cellulite.

3

JULY 14, 1996
JUSTICE DEPARTMENT BUILDING, WASHINGTON, D.C.

This can't be right. It's the sub-basement! thought Vida Johnson as she stepped out of the elevator at FBI headquarters. But this was where the man in the lobby had directed her. A long, dimly lit corridor stretched before her, water pipes and heating ducts running the length of its ceiling. She felt her nerves tighten, automatically tying a knot in her belly. This was going to be much worse than she had imagined. She had expected merely government-issue dreadful. That would have been a treat in comparison to this.

Vida looked around, somewhat stunned, completely out of place in these surroundings. Her light blue summer dress was incongruous against the drab institutional gray walls, but she looked breathtakingly beautiful in the stark bare-bulb light of the corridor. Delicate, yet strangely powerful. An interesting paradox. But there was no one to appreciate the effect: FBI Agent Vida Johnson standing alone, a solitary black woman squaring her shoulders before a very hostile world.

An arrow-shaped sign on the wall indicated that the morgue was to her right. She'd been instructed to head in the other direction. That seemed like a positive omen. Vida passed one doorway marked Furnace Room and several others that were unmarked. Then the corridor made a sharp right turn. In a cul-de-sac about a hundred feet in front of her was an open doorway with light blue smoke lazily curling out. Vida approached it.

Inside, all she could see was his back. The pitifully cramped room was dark except for a desk lamp. He was hunched over the desk, his head wreathed in thick blue smoke. Vida cleared her throat with authority and asked, "Agent Levitt?" in a much smaller voice than she had rehearsed in her head.

The man turned his head toward the door, straightened up, rose out of his seat, and kept on rising until he nearly filled the smoky room with his presence. Vida took a nervous step back from the door. Lord, she couldn't remember ever having seen such a huge white man. His stepping into the lighted hallway didn't diminish the impression. He stared down at her from a great height, drinking in a first impression. Vida returned the appraising look as steadfastly as she could.

This Levitt person had to be six-five and weigh close to 290 pounds. Vida judged him to be in his midfifties. What she could see of his hair appeared to be black, thinning and going gray. He had an unruly walruslike mustache and a thick, really foul-smelling stogie sticking out of his mouth. Agent Levitt had a plaster cast on his left forearm, with only the fingers poking out one end.

But the giant flashed a warm smile and said, "You must be Agent Johnson. Welcome to Siberia!"

Without another word he dropped his cigar on the floor, stomped on it with a size 13 gunboat of a shoe, turned to his desk, and began to fan the air with a file folder. "Sorry about the smog. I'll have to stop smoking down here now that you've been assigned to the area."

Vida felt herself bristle. "You mean this is my office?"

The giant shook his head rather apologetically and said, "Afraid not. It's *our* office."

Vida peered into the darkened niche. The large desk nearly filled a room that surely must have been a janitor's station at one time. What space remained was filled to capacity with metal shelves overflowing with folders and books. There was a single chair in which Agent Ira Levitt was graciously motioning her to sit. Vida decided that perhaps this was a good idea. The ludicrousness of the situation was liable to hit her at any moment. It would be best to be seated when it did.

Ira drew back into the room, wedged himself into one corner, and perched there on the edge of the desk. He was watching every nuance of Vida's reaction. "Not exactly what you expected, eh?"

"Not even close."

Vida struggled with her irritation as the giant shifted his weight. Finally he crossed his arms and said, "Let's start off right. Okay? I know all about your prior experience with the Bureau. I'm not overjoyed about your being assigned to me, but not for the reasons you might think."

Agent Johnson rubbed her forehead, certain she knew what was coming.

Ira picked up a file and thumbed through it. "They sent me your personnel file. I read about your trouble with Richard Davenport, at least the official version. But I don't like to depend on one source for any kind of information, so I called around Baltimore and got the straight poop."

Vida's face registered her surprise. He continued without giving her a chance to speak. "Davenport hit on you for six months, trying to get you between the sheets. He wasn't exactly subtle about it. Everyone in the office knew what was going on."

"Pity none of those guys had the guts to testify on my behalf at the hearing. When push came to shove, it was my word against his."

Ira nodded. "They understand that Davenport's extremely well connected politically. Hell, they weren't going to stick their necks out for someone they hardly knew. The consensus is that you pretty well went it alone in Baltimore. So when you got in trouble with Davenport you had no one to turn to for help. You had to conceal a tape recorder on your person to get evidence for the review board. Nice piece of work, that."

Vida caught Ira smiling at her. "I had no choice. That bastard Davenport finally said flat out that if I didn't sleep with him he'd turn in the worst quarterly performance evaluation any agent ever saw. So I hired an attorney. He took a copy of the recording to Davenport's superiors."

Ira tossed the file on the desk and resumed his recitation. "That got Davenport a letter of censure in his service record and a transfer to Utah. Coincidentally, two weeks later you were informed that you were being transferred. They probably assured you six ways from Sunday that your transfer had absolutely nothing to do with the Davenport affair. Am I right?"

Vida thoughtfully chewed her lower lip and then, deciding she had nothing to lose, said, "I never believed it for a second. They claimed their manpower quotas had been cut, and since I was the junior agent in the office . . . Everyone kept telling me how Washington was a great place to be posted and how much I'd love it. Am I going to love it?"

"I doubt it. This department is where they send the unrepentant and the unwanted."

"Is that why you're here?"

Ira grinned maniacally at this question, and Vida was sorry she'd asked. It felt like a setup.

"You got it. I'm here because I'm the king of the fuckups. Crown Prince Schmegegi. See, there was this Christmas office party in 1978 at which my supervisor got tanked and took a swing at me. Being a little juiced myself, I guess I overreacted a bit. I broke the jerk's jaw. Fortunately there were plenty of witnesses, so I was cleared at the disciplinary hearing. But wouldn't you know it? A month later I was transferred down here, and I've been here ever since. Do you have any idea who that supervisor was?"

"No."

"His name was Richard Davenport. Now, I tell you this story for two reasons, neither of them a desire to elicit sympathy. You better realize a couple of things right now. In six months Davenport will probably be transferred back to Baltimore, all sins forgiven. You, on the other hand, will never get a reprieve as long as Davenport's in the Bureau. You crossed one of the biggest old boys in the old boy network. That transgression will never be forgotten.

"The other reason I've told you how I came by this elevated position is so you don't misunderstand my resistance to your being assigned to me. Believe me, it has nothing to do with the crap Davenport put you through.

"Your records show that nearly all your experience with the Bureau has been clerical. No fieldwork, no arrests. I'm working on a tough investigation, tracking down a serial murderer. That's how I got this broken wing you've so tactfully neglected to mention."

Vida calmly gazed at Ira and said, "If you look further through my records, you'll find I have a marksmanship rating with a .38 caliber automatic and that I'm in excellent physical shape. I run three miles each morning before breakfast and have a brown belt in karate. I've applied for field duty several times during my two years with the Bureau. The requests were turned down by Richard Davenport. It's true that I have no field experience, but I'll never get any if my superiors keep holding the lack of it against me."

Ira eased his bulk off the desk, his expression thoughtful. When he reached the door, he said noncommittally over his shoulder, "Well, maybe we can work something out. Let's take a walk. I spend as little time here as possible. Oh, and don't bother trying to lock up. The door's busted. Been that way as long as I can remember. Nothing in here worth stealing anyway."

Ira and Vida climbed the side stairs and went out through a fire door. Neither said a word until they found themselves wandering down Pennsylvania Avenue. Vida was the one to break the prolonged silence. "This multiple homicide you're working on—what's the Bureau's interest in it?"

"The murders have taken place in several different states, so the Bureau decided to step in. Officially you and

I are assigned to the Major Crimes Division. Even though it has received no publicity, the Bureau considers this weird case a nasty one. Messy. Very messy. And one that could backfire at any time, proving a real embarrassment politically for any number of big *machers* in the old boy network. Secretly the Bureau wishes it had never gotten involved. They jumped in before getting the whole picture. That's why they made it my headache. If it goes sour, they'll blame it all on me. I've been investigating it from the beginning."

"How long has it been an open case?"

"Seven years next month."

Vida let this sink in for a moment, then asked, "How many people has he killed?"

"Eighteen."

"He's killed eighteen people and we're the only two agents assigned to the case?"

"Hell, you wouldn't have even been put on the job if I hadn't gotten myself tagged last month. The Bureau doesn't take kindly to wanted felons going around clubbing its agents senseless, even the unloved ones."

"You seem to have left something out, Agent Levitt."

"Call me Ira."

"An interstate murder case of this magnitude should have a major task force trying to crack it."

"I can see this is going to take some serious explaining," said Ira, half lost in thought. Then he brightened visibly. "Say, you like Mexican food?"

"Uh, sure."

"Then I suggest we have us an early lunch, over which I'll tell you the saga of David Vandemark, the most fascinating murderer I've had the misfortune to track."

4

JULY 1996
SANIBEL, FLORIDA

Six strangers sitting around a poker table in room 415 of the Royal Palms Hotel. Four lambs and two wolves. Not exactly the setup Roger Cordell had had in mind originally, yet he felt confidently in control of the situation. He adjusted his rose-tinted sunglasses on the bridge of his nose as he scanned the table.

To Roger's left was Peter Midler. Roger had met him on the beach earlier in the week. Peter had looked rather forlorn playing solitaire on his blanket while his wife and kids frolicked in the surf. Ever on the lookout for a likely prospect, Roger had struck up a conversation and soon discovered that Midler was an insurance executive from Chicago with a secret passion for high-stakes poker. Roger found it child's play to wrangle an invitation to the next game.

The timing had been perfect. Roger was down to his last five hundred dollars, and he knew from experience that a game of poker was the easiest way to replenish his dwindling resources. His gift conveniently took all the chance out of that game.

Next to Pete Midler sat Sol Perlman, a divorced stockbroker from New York. Solly thought the best way to spend his holiday away from Wall Street was to hole up in his Florida hotel room for two weeks playing cards. These were his digs.

Directly across the table from Roger was Art Benedict, a large, balding black man. Benedict was the richest of the four sheep, owner of a chain of grocery stores in Milwaukee. But this was something he didn't bring up in the table talk. He was content to simply have everyone in the game think of him as just another harried small businessman, trying to get away from it all. The only reason he was there, really, was to kill a few hours. He was waiting to meet the late-night flight that was bringing the rest of his family in from Chicago. Can't wait to see 'em, Art thought. Sure miss 'em all. Yes sir, especially my Lucille.

To Art's left was Mike Klairmont, owner of a huge Nissan dealership in Pittsburgh. He'd come to Florida to hobnob with rich folks so he could feel important when he went home next week. So far the vacation had been a total washout. All those glittering private parties aboard obscenely large yachts had somehow managed to elude him. Roger was highly amused by Klairmont's inflated sense of self-worth, not to mention his rather tenuous grasp on reality.

Four sheep come to be clipped. They would have been horrified if they'd realized how much Roger knew about them. Luckily for them, Roger had decided to leave these lambs unsheared. In fact, the only person at the table Roger had any interest in was the man sitting to his right, the other wolf. Olive-skinned, with piercing dark eyes, he claimed his name was Dominic Sanchez and that he owned a hotel in Mexico.

Only Roger knew it was a lie.

Dominic's last name was actually Torres, and he was from Bogotá, Colombia. He did own a hotel in Costa Rica, from which he ran a string of prostitutes, but even that was a sideline for him. Dominic's main source of income was cocaine. Roger also knew that the slab of beef sitting in the kitchenette sipping a beer wasn't really Dominic's cousin Isidro, a big harmless slob with nothing to do—"Let him sit in the kitchen, reading his paper. He won't bother us." Big-time drug smugglers like Dominic never went anywhere without their bodyguards.

Quite suddenly this quiet little fleecing had become something else entirely. Roger cursed himself roundly for not having had the foresight to bring some firepower along, especially since he had a small arsenal stashed in the trunk of his rental car. A hell of a lot of good it would do him sitting in the hotel parking lot, baking in the sun. Anyway, how was he supposed to know he'd have to kill someone that afternoon? He hadn't planned this. But one look into Dominic's mind had changed everything. He would have to execute this man. There was no getting around it.

⨯⨯⨯

Usually Roger followed five rules at these poker benefits, as he liked to call them. Rule number one: Never take more than the mark can afford to lose. Hurt feelings were all right, but Roger didn't want to ruin anyone's life while enriching himself. Number two: If the cards are going your way, take only every third hand, after building the pot up to a more than respectable level. It looks a tad suspicious when you take nearly every one. Three: Let the

game go on as long as you can. That way all players leave
the table tired, feeling they've given it their all. Four:
Never abuse another player's ego while emptying his
pockets. Let the loser walk away with his dignity. Five:
Spread the loss across the table as evenly as possible.
Never set up any one person as the main contributor.

Following these rules had allowed Roger to waltz away
the winner in over a hundred big-money games without
ever having to defend himself against a violent loser. But
Roger had never played cards with a man like Dominic
Torres before. So rules four and five went right out the
window. Roger rolled up his sleeves and went to work on
the Colombian.

∽∾∽∾

The Royal Palms Hotel was one of Sanibel's more luxurious tourist traps: $400 a night, all glass and chrome,
wall-to-wall mirrors in the bedrooms. Las Vegas–style os-
tentation. Needless to say, everyone but Roger was staying here.

Roger made sure that all of the participants except Dominic stayed about even. That wasn't hard to do, since
Roger was in effect playing five of the six hands. No need
even to mark the cards.

One hour into the game, Dominic was down $12,000,
give or take a couple hundred. At this point the other
players, including Roger, tried to talk the Colombian into
calling it a day. The cards weren't being kind to him, they
said, and Roger couldn't resist adding that perhaps poker
might be unsuited to the Latin American's temperament.

His machismo challenged, Dominic steadfastly refused to quit. Thirty minutes later he was $18,000 in the hole.

The dope dealer kept fishing into his money belt, producing seemingly endless fresh rolls of crisp hundred-dollar bills, as Roger egged him on. Still playing the obnoxious American, Cordell kept assuring Dominic that sooner or later he would get the hang of the game, though he knew it could not have escaped Dominic's attention that most of his money was sitting in front of Cordell, the computer programmer from Detroit.

When Roger had accumulated more than $23,000 of Dominic's ill-gotten fortune, he decided it was time to call it quits. He borrowed Dominic's gold lighter to fire up a cigarette and now sat at the table staring at it. Everyone at the game thought Roger was daydreaming. None of them could have guessed that he was actually engaging in a bit of psychotelemetry: the trace impressions on the lighter revealed volumes about its owner.

Out of patience, Dominic grabbed the lighter from Roger's hand. "We going to play cards or what, man?" he demanded.

It was Roger's deal. Pete handed him the deck. Roger smiled broadly as he shuffled the cards, his eyes locked on Dominic's. This brazen test of wills had the desired effect on the Colombian's frayed nerves.

"What are you looking at, *maricón?*" said Dominic in his best fuck-you voice. "You got a problem?"

Roger donned his most bored expression. "No, I was just sitting here wondering what the weather in Bogotá must be like this time of year."

Roger couldn't have gotten a more satisfying reaction if

he had poured hot coffee into Dominic's lap. The dope dealer stiffened and glared at him. "How would I know?"

The smile on Roger's face broadened. "I wasn't asking, Dom. I was just wondering out loud. Looks like the subject bothers you a bit, though. How come?"

"It don't bother me. I thought you were asking me a question, that's all."

Roger nodded and announced the game to be seven-card stud as he dealt out the first three cards to each player, one down, two up. Sol Perlman wound up with a king and ten showing, and he kicked off the betting at $100. Roger upped it to $200 when it came around. As he dealt out the fourth card, Roger glanced over at Dominic and said, "I've got it! Now I remember where I saw your cousin Isidro before. He was a professional wrestler in Mexico, wasn't he? I spent a little time down there a few years back. Say, didn't Isidro break someone's back and lose his license?"

The slab of beef in the kitchenette stirred restlessly, his interest in the newspaper having evaporated instantly. Dominic flashed him a warning glance and signaled with a slight shake of his head that he had the situation under control. Then he turned back to Roger and, in exaggeratedly precise English, said, "You're quite right about that, Mr. Cordell. You must have a good memory for faces. A terrible misfortune befell Isidro, you understand? Such things happen in professional sports. I had him come to work for me because he can no longer pursue his chosen career."

Roger looked appropriately sympathetic to Isidro's dilemma as he upped Perlman's bet from $200 to $400 on the second go-around. "Well, that was mighty nice of you, bringing your cousin into your import business when his luck went south."

Dominic got an ugly look on his face. Cousin Isidro silently rose out of his chair. Only Roger noticed. Dominic leaned toward Roger menacingly as he said, "Hotel business."

"Oh, sure. My mistake."

Roger flipped each player a fifth card. Sol, with two kings showing, broke fast out of the gate with a $500 bet. "Feeling lucky this hand!" he said. Pete Midler folded. Roger doubled the bet. Dominic eyed the dealer suspiciously but decided to see the bet anyway. Both Mike Klairmont and Art Benedict disgustedly threw in their cards. "Too rich," Klairmont grumbled. Sol decided to hang in there, hoping to come up with a pair to go with his three kings.

As Roger dealt the sixth card to the remaining players, he remarked, "Say, Dominic, you ever hear of another Dominic, a guy named Torres?"

Torres didn't move a muscle. He sat there like a statue, frozen in the act of examining his hole card. A full ten seconds later, ten seconds during which time seemed to slow to a standstill, he let the card drop back onto the table and said, "No, why do you ask?"

Sol bet another $500, and Roger raised it to $1,000 before answering Dominic's question. "You look a lot like this Torres character. He's a coke dealer from Bogotá."

Dominic tossed his thousand dollars' worth of chips into the pot without a word. Sol Perlman abruptly folded. The sheep were suddenly intensely aware of the wolves in their midst. Every eye at the table was on Dominic and Roger as Isidro stepped up behind Solly. The flock was nervous, excruciatingly aware of the threat posed by Isidro's massive presence.

Cordell smiled at Dominic and inquired cheerfully, "Up or down?"

"Down."

Roger flipped one last card to Dominic, then dealt himself one. As each man looked at his hole card, the Colombian spoke, his voice steady and as smooth as silk. "You are not who you pretend to be, are you, Mr. Cordell? Who are you, really?"

"Not DEA, if that's what you're worried about. I work for myself, not Uncle Sam. Strictly freelance."

"Then what do you want from me?"

"To start with, I'd like to see your hole cards."

"That, Señor Cordell, will cost you."

Dominic flipped three thousand dollars' worth of chips onto the center of the table. Roger did the same and called. The Colombian slowly and theatrically turned over his two hole cards, one at a time, revealing a total of four slyly smiling ladies. He let his right hand drift to his lap. Roger knew Dominic was inching his way to the derringer strapped to his calf. Roger pretended to be oblivious to the danger. Meanwhile, Isidro shifted his position, which put him directly behind an increasingly anxious Peter Midler.

Taking his cue from Dominic, Roger, with great ceremony, turned his hole cards over, one at a time, until his straight flush lay face up.

Dominic cleared his throat. The clean, crisp, deadly voice said, "You have received your first wish, my friend. You perhaps want something else from me?"

"I'd like to ask you a question."

"Then maybe we should leave these gentlemen to their game and talk privately."

"No, I like it here just fine. It doesn't matter to me if they hear what we say."

Dominic glanced coolly around the room, then shrugged. "Very well. Ask your question, señor, but I cannot guarantee you will like my answer."

"That hardly matters now," Roger said as he leaned closer to Dominic. The Colombian did likewise, thinking the movement would hide his hand closing around the grip of the derringer. Their faces were only inches apart when Roger said, "I know the first two were just business, a couple of rival dealers trying to muscle in on your territory. And I realize that the two DEA agents had to die because they were going to cost you money by interrupting the smooth flow of your supply lines. Those four deaths I understand. But why did you kill Sandra Cruz the way you did?"

Roger paused to look around the table. Nobody breathed. Even the gigantic Isidro seemed frozen as he listened.

Roger decided to press his advantage. "Sandra was a nineteen-year-old girl living in Bogotá when Dominic first met her," he said. "She was poor and not exactly a Rhodes scholar, so she was impressed by Dominic's flashy clothes, big cars, and fancy home. After she moved into his house in Miami it took her six months to figure out that Dominic wasn't an investment banker, as he claimed to be. See, the fellow has this bad habit of lying about his occupation. I can understand why.

"Unfortunately Sandra had read way too many romance novels. She'd bought in to the idea that a good woman could save her man if she really put her mind to it, or maybe her heart. Sandra begged Dom to quit the drug game and settle down into some honest business. His answer was to lock her in a room and get her hooked on heroin. That kept her in line for a while. But then she found out that he'd murdered two DEA agents, and she got spooked."

Roger turned back toward Dominic and smiled into the man's expressionless face.

"You had to hustle her onto the yacht and split from Miami before she spilled her guts. That's when you and Isidro did her, on the trip back to Colombia.

"But it was different with Sandra, wasn't it? This time you killed for fun. It gave you a real rush. You got your goon to wire an anchor to her ankles. Then you had Isidro throw her overboard. You still get excited when you remember the expression on her face as she hit the water, don't you?"

Roger let Dominic bring the gun all the way up from under the table before he slammed a fist into the Colombian's throat. He felt something snap under the impact. Dominic sputtered, choked, and dropped the derringer onto the table as he crumpled to the floor.

Isidro lunged forward, and Roger spun to face him. As the approaching giant made a grab for him, Cordell latched on to the wrestler's huge right thumb with his left hand, then jammed the thumb of his other hand between the knuckles of Isidro's third finger and pinkie and slammed the behemoth face down onto the card table. As the table tipped over onto the strangling Dominic, Roger seized the derringer.

Isidro, his nose bleeding, was back on his feet in a flash, charging toward Roger, his thick arms reaching out to crush and mangle. Roger fired once. The bullet ripped into Isidro's kneecap, shattering it. Isidro Fortaleza, once known as El Hombre Montaña, went down moaning, grasping his ruined knee. With Roger blocking the only exit, the sheep sought sanctuary behind the bed and in the bathroom.

Meanwhile Dominic, lying on the floor next to Isidro, began to spasm, his oxygen-starved brain sending out chaotic signals to the rest of his body. Roger thought his movements looked a little like a dance of penance and death.

Roger stepped over to the vase that had served as the bank and dumped its contents onto the floor. He collected what he calculated to be his winnings and pocketed them. By that time Dominic had quit thrashing. From the relative safety of their protected vantage points, the sheep had watched Dominic's end, numbly mute in their fascination with his death throes.

Isidro rolled over and committed to memory every detail of the man who had just hobbled him, so that he might one day kill him. Roger let Isidro get a good look.

"Guess it's been a hard day for you, Isidro. Unemployed and crippled all in the same afternoon. Looks like you'll be searching for a new career—again. *Que lástima.*"

Isidro spit in Roger's general direction. *"Hijo de puta!"*

Allowing only a slight twitch of the jaw in response, Roger nodded his approval of the wrestler's bravado, then stepped forward and emptied the derringer's second chamber into Isidro's forehead. The giant let out a groan and rolled face down.

The man who had been David Vandemark turned and strolled out of the hotel. No one tried to stop him. As he made his way across the parking lot, he sighed rather sadly; it looked as if his vacation was over. Time to say farewell to sunny Sanibel.

5

They were sitting at a table in the "outdoor" cafe, which was hermetically sealed against the heat and humidity. Vida selected a house salad while Ira ordered what seemed like a quarter of the menu. The obsequious treatment they'd received from the staff was beginning to make sense. Ira Levitt was evidently one of this establishment's most valued customers.

The burly FBI agent had put Vida off until now, claiming that he was unable to talk about David Vandemark on an empty stomach. Though Vida didn't buy Ira's explanation, she was beginning to understand that her new partner had his own ways of doing things and that she would have to get used to them.

On the walk to the restaurant, Ira had learned that Vida was single, that she attended law school at night, and that she had three younger brothers and a mother at home. In return, he had volunteered that he'd been divorced for nearly ten years, but little else. Vida got the impression that he wasn't being closemouthed or evasive about his personal life. He simply had none. She'd met other agents whose total existence revolved around the Bureau. In Ira's case this seemed doubly tragic. A mental picture of the basement office at the Federal Building made Vida shudder.

By the time the waiter returned with her club soda and Ira's bottle of Dos Equis, Vida's patience was nearly depleted. She allowed him one quick sip of his beer. Then she prodded him: "Well, tell me about Vandemark."

Ira noted her impatience with a gentle amusement, took another sip of his beer, and said simply, "He was a corporate lawyer, out in Michigan."

"You're kidding, right?"

"Nope."

"A serial murderer who used to be a lawyer?"

"Damn good one too, from what I've been able to gather. The senior partners at his law firm, Bradhurt, Weiss, and Lowe, were the first people I interviewed when I started my background check. For three years Vandemark worked at the Bloomfield Hills office of this prestigious firm, where he established a reputation as a perfectionist and workaholic. Everyone assumed he'd make senior partner before the third year was up. Vandemark was a real hotshot. Married Lowe's daughter. Perfect embodiment of a man rapidly ascending the legal ladder of success."

Dandy, just dandy, thought Vida, the part-time law student. This coincidence was a little too weird. Her first multiple murderer, and he turns out to be an attorney. This day was shaping up to be a real winner. She touched her temple lightly, an unconscious gesture in anticipation of the headache she was sure she'd be going home with at the end of the day.

"Back in 1989," Ira continued, "Detroit was going through a boom that pushed property values up through the roof, especially in the area near the Renaissance Center. Most of the firm's clients were Detroit Realtors and developers."

"I see. Vandemark was an ambitious yuppie lawyer making his bones in the firm."

Ira scratched his chin as he mulled over Vida's comment. "I guess you could say that. Vandemark had a keen legal mind. Brought in a lot of bucks for the firm. He was their fair-haired boy. But you see, he refused to compromise his high ethical standards. More than once, apparently, he talked his clients into coughing up extra cash to relocate the poor people his firm helped evict. There was a lot of that going on in Detroit at the time. Big-time real estate interests muscled every mom-and-pop store out of the area.

"Vandemark did his share of that dirty work, but he was a bit more humane about it than most. He also did quite a bit of pro bono work for folks who couldn't afford a lawyer. His bosses' only gripe was this tendency to favor the underdog, but they were sure a couple more years with the firm would work that completely out of his system. Of course, they never got a chance to test their theory."

"What happened?"

"There was an accident. Then the murder. But I'm getting ahead of myself. I'd better fill you in on the background before I jump into the heart of the matter."

Before Ira could continue, the waiter placed a double order of nachos in front of him. Ira made the proper gustatory exclamations, nodded his approval to the beaming waiter, and dived into the hearty fare. Munching made Ira philosophical. "You know, I think if Vandemark hadn't gotten himself trapped in his pursuit of the American Dream, he might've made one hell of a civil rights lawyer. But he had a wife and kid to support, and a mortgaged house in the suburbs."

"What was his family life like?"

"Let me tell you, it was the kind of family Norman Rockwell loved to paint. Christine Vandemark was a radiant flaxen-haired beauty. Down to earth despite her patrician good looks, her family's considerable new money, and social standing. She used to be a schoolteacher, and she was planning to go back to teaching when their daughter got older. By all accounts, David Vandemark absolutely adored her. She apparently felt the same way about him.

"Their little girl, Jennifer, was only four years old when it happened." Ira stopped for a second, his voice full of regret. "Pretty little thing. Took after her mother. The resemblance was striking in the photos I saw."

From the rather intimate way he spoke of them, Vida had surmised he'd been talking about people he'd actually known. "You never met the mother or child?"

Ira took a deep swallow of beer without looking up. "Not while they were alive."

Her next question died stillborn on Vida's lips. After a moment of silence, Ira plunged back into his narrative. "The three of them lived in a three-bedroom house in Warren, Michigan, a quiet little suburb; big backyard, grade school down the street. They planned to move to a larger place once David got his promotion."

Ira's attention was drawn to something outside the window. Vida followed his gaze and spotted a young couple walking down the street with two blond boys in tow. Ira continued to watch them wander out of sight as he said, "At first I thought the key to why David committed the murders might have been hidden somewhere in his family life. That turned out to be a dead end. The Vandemarks were a model couple: loving, healthy, their whole wonderful lives ahead of them. Or so it must have seemed. They couldn't have been happier."

"How about his life before he got married?" Vida asked.

"High school, law school, met his wife in college, married her after he passed the bar exam. Everything exactly as it was supposed to be. No surprises. The only unusual thing about his past, in fact, was that he'd been raised by an aunt. Supposedly his parents were killed in an auto accident in Ohio, but I found out this was a crock of shit."

Once more the waiter interrupted Ira's story, this time to bring Vida's salad and Ira's cornucopia of Mexican delights. Ooh, child, if that ain't a wallow in pig heaven I don't know what is, Vida thought as she looked across the table at the mammoth collection of burritos, enchiladas, tacos, rice, and refried beans. She glumly examined her salad. "So anyway, what ended this blissful existence?"

Ira's reply was muffled by a mouthful of enchilada. "The accident. It sounded pretty horrible from the reports I've read. Two people died."

"Vandemark's wife and child?"

"No. One of them was a real estate developer named Joseph Scarpelli. The other was a contractor called Mullaney or Malone—I forget. Some kind of Irish name. Not important."

"I daresay it was to him." Ira seemed not to hear this. "A car accident, you say?" Vida prompted.

"I didn't say. No, it was an elevator accident. An ancient, dilapidated elevator. Almost killed him, Vandemark. Probably should have. It would have been better for everyone if it had."

6

MIAMI

Before dropping his car off at the rental office, Willard MacDonald slit the lining of his suitcase with a pocketknife. Within lay all the documentation he needed to prove that this blond, bearded gentleman was truly who he claimed to be, an air traffic controller from Boston.

Willard felt bad about having had to leave all his colorful Hawaiian shirts back at the Snook Motel, along with the snappy little Walther P-38 that was stashed under the mattress of the room's extra bed. He hadn't wasted time going back to the motel. He knew that Torres's murder would have local authorities shutting Sanibel Island down tight as a drum. He had no intention of cutting this any closer than he had to, so he'd headed for the Sanibel Causeway immediately after the killing and kept right on going. Three hours of driving east on Alligator Alley, U.S. 41, had brought him into Miami.

He'd arrived as the sun began to set at his back. Enough time left to turn in the rental car before catching the early-evening train north, a red-eye that would reach New York City at 7:39 the following morning. No more airlines for Willard, at least not until he'd worked out a way to get past airport security metal detectors without setting off the alarms. That bullet in his leg had turned out to be something of a problem after all.

Willard breathed a sigh of relief when he found there was a sleeper available. He'd been afraid that he'd have to fold himself uncomfortably into one of those double seats in the passenger section. It would have played havoc with his mending leg.

Noticing Willard's limp, a porter offered to help him with his bag. Mr. MacDonald graciously declined, explaining that his doctor had ordered him to exercise the damn leg; that was the only way it was going to get any better. Besides, the suitcase wasn't nearly as heavy as it looked.

That was a lie. The porter would probably have gotten a hernia trying to carry Willard's bag. It contained two .38 caliber Smith & Wesson automatics, a 9 mm 16-round Beretta, an Uzi machine pistol with enough ammunition to hold off a battalion of marines, a shaving kit, and two changes of clothing. This was Willard's idea of traveling light. Another good reason to avoid airport security.

Willard tossed off a friendly smile in the general direction of the conscientious porter, gritted his teeth, lifted his bag, and headed for the loading platform. The pain in his leg was excruciating. He'd nearly passed out twice as he walked across the parking lot to the station. Willard had to pause three more times to rest in order to reach his train. A good-natured, well-built young sailor, heading home on leave, helped Willard get the bag onto the train, but at a cost. He wanted to know what was so damn heavy inside the suitcase. Rocks? Willard immediately jumped into a monologue about how he'd promised all his friends in Crab Apple Cove, New Hampshire, a bottle of Florida sand when he came back from his vacation. He'd only gotten through the names and personal histories of three of his exceedingly dull fictitious friends when the swabbie excused himself, claiming an urgent call of nature.

Willard found his compartment without further difficulty, stowed his suitcase, and sat down on the edge of the room's already unfolded bed. Its siren call was almost too much for him to resist. But Willard decided he'd better stay awake and on guard until the train left the station.

Looking out the window, he allowed his thoughts to turn to something that had been nagging at him since he first walked into room 415 of the Royal Palms Hotel and laid eyes on Dominic Torres. Everything had been happening so fast that he hadn't had time to inspect the nagging thought. But now, alone and safe in the sanctuary of this private compartment, he could examine the mental irritant that had been rolling around the periphery of his consciousness like a pebble in a shoe for the past five hours.

Dominic had reminded him of someone else. But for the life of him, the newly minted Mr. Willard MacDonald couldn't remember who that someone was.

He told himself not to push it. Watch the busy people hustling by outside the window. The name would float to the surface in due time.

The train abruptly lurched into motion as the answer to his question dawned on him. Willard smiled at the recollection. Of course. Like Dominic, another nasty little shit. Both of them had black hair and bad dispositions. And both probably deserved to die. God, had it been seven years already?

As Willard's mind revisited a different world in a comfortable little house in the suburb of Warren, Michigan, in 1989, his lips spoke the name: "Joseph Scarpelli."

7

MAY 21, 1989
WARREN, MICHIGAN

David Vandemark lay in bed, savoring the drowsiness that lingered along his awareness. Sleeping late was a treat he'd been denied for some time, so he was thoroughly enjoying himself as he alternated between bouts of napping and moments of semi-wakefulness.

He tried to fend off total consciousness as long as possible, but the happily intrusive sounds of his daughter, Jennifer, were drifting in through the open window of their upstairs bedroom. Judging by the war whoops, she was playing on the swing set he'd put up in the yard. The swings were a big hit with her, but Jenny's gleeful enjoyment of them had shattered more than one morning's slumber. He rolled over, one eye open, and saw that the clock on the nightstand read 10:47 A.M. Well, he'd managed to get in over ten hours of nap time. That was certainly enough, but he could have kept snoozing endlessly. David had been working entirely too hard of late. Burning the candle at both ends was beginning to catch up with him.

He remained in bed, staring up at the ceiling and thinking about work. That was the way it always seemed to be lately. As soon as a clear thought could form in the morning, it was usually about the job. David didn't like this realization or its implications. This was surely one of the early-warning signs of workaholism.

Feeling slightly annoyed with himself, David slung his legs over the side of the bed, got up, and headed for the bathroom, pausing at the full-length mirror on the door long enough to take inventory. He wasn't at all certain he liked the image that stared back. His light brown hair hadn't turned gray or fallen out since the last time he looked, and he had not become stoop-shouldered or obese. But the twenty-six-year-old, five-foot-eleven-inch guy in the mirror somehow wasn't quite the man David remembered. There was a puffiness around his eyes that shouldn't have been there, a recent development. And the once clearly defined stomach muscles had begun to let gravity have its way with them. He hadn't gone to fat, mind you, he'd only lost some of his tautness. A little time at the gym would remedy that. David smiled both at his male vanity and at his duplicitous nature. He knew it didn't matter if he was getting a teeny bit soft around the middle. He'd never find the time to get to the gym. It had been six months at least since he'd been there; his membership had probably lapsed. The job was taking over his life lately. There was precious little time for anything else.

It wouldn't have been so bad if he'd been doing something he enjoyed. But it had been ages since David's work had included anything more challenging than writing and vetting contracts and dealing with contractors on behalf of the firm's clients. He was beginning to forget what the inside of a courtroom looked like. David pined for a vagrancy or assault charge to defend. A murder was surely too much to hope for.

I know, he thought as he stepped into the shower. If wishes were horses, beggars would ride.

He had no idea that this was the last day of his life.

❧❧❧

David found Christine in the kitchen. She had a morning kiss and a cup of coffee waiting for him. He caught a faint hint of her perfume as they disengaged. The fragrance triggered memories of their lovemaking the night before. He sat down at the kitchen counter and smiled as he watched Chris sashay over to the refrigerator.

Over her shoulder she said, "What sounds good for breakfast? I've got some Canadian bacon . . ."

"Sure, and a couple of scrambled eggs. Oh, and keep the coffee flowing."

"I was beginning to think you'd never get up, Dave."

David grinned at her lasciviously. "Funny, that's not what you said last night."

"You're a bad boy, David."

Chris danced over to him, bacon in hand, gave him a kiss on the nape of the neck and a pinch on the back of something else. David swiveled around on the bar stool, but his wife had already made her escape.

As she cracked two eggs into a bowl, she said, "I think last night qualified you for the *Guinness Book of World Records*, baby. I was afraid we were going to wake Jenny."

"Wouldn't matter, she's four. Old enough to know Mommy and Daddy do strange and wonderful things to each other behind their closed bedroom door."

They drifted into an easy silence while Christine busied herself with breakfast and David tried to piece together the remnants of that morning's *Detroit Free Press*. What am I going to do with you, Chris? he thought indulgently. Even after five years of marriage he hadn't been able to break Christine of her habit of disemboweling the paper so she could read it easily while working around the house. It never occurred to her to reassemble it afterward. No use complaining about this aberrant behavioral trait. Whenever he brought the subject up, Chris promised to mend her ways only to return to them with renewed gusto the very next day. Some battles were not meant to be won, and David had resigned himself to learning the day's news in scattered bits and pieces.

After finding out that the Tigers had blown last night's game in extra innings, David gazed out the kitchen window at Jennifer and her friend from down the street. What was the little girl's name? Kathy? Karen? Well, never mind . . . The kids had abandoned the swing set for considerably more tactile pleasures. They were busy making a mess of themselves in the sandbox. It had rained the day before and both girls were thoroughly caked with sticky sand. No reason to ruin their fun by telling Mom about it prematurely. There'd be hell to pay, but it could wait. David was enjoying Christine's presence too much to send her off on a disciplinary mission.

Glancing around, David decided all the long hours and hard work were worth it. He was more than satisfied with his lot in life. He had a beautiful blond wife, whom he had never even thought about cheating on, and a lovely daughter who was a perfect blending of the best of himself and Christine—except when she was misbehaving, of course. But that was much less often since she had reached the mature, reasonable age of four.

They would live happily in their comfy three-bedroom home, at least until their urge to be fruitful and multiply drove them to seek a larger dwelling. The game plan called for a new home closer to the office. But that change would have to wait until he became a full partner and could afford one of those sprawling high-priced houses in Bloomfield Hills. Maybe then he would be able to get back to the kind of law he wanted to practice. In the meantime, there were dues to be paid.

Christine placed David's breakfast before him and sat down at the counter beside him, a cup of coffee in hand.

"We on for the Runstroms' tonight?" she asked, settling in.

"Sure, I'm in the mood for a party. I'll be finished painting the trim on the garage and cleaned up by five."

"Jesus, I almost forgot!"

David knew what that meant. "I got a call while I was asleep, right?"

Chris gave David a heartfelt look of sympathy before answering. "Daddy called and said Mr. Muldoon would meet you at the plant on Cass Avenue at one o'clock this afternoon."

"Christ Almighty! That asshole Muldoon's been ducking my calls all week and now he wants me to hoof it downtown to meet him on my day off? Sorry, pal, it doesn't work that way. He can wait till Monday."

"That's what I told Daddy, but it turns out Muldoon's flying to Chicago on Monday. The bank wants to see Mr. Muldoon's cost estimates for the renovation work before they'll approve Mr. Scarpelli's loan. If you don't take care of it today, the deal could be jeopardized."

Marrying the boss's daughter was decidedly a double-edged sword. David had been fortunate that his wife didn't consider his job a rival. Her father, Vincent Lowe of Bradhurst, Weiss, and Lowe, had taught his daughter that the law firm was an integral part of their family life. Christine and her brother, Tom, had never questioned or rebelled against the circumstance. Each had made choices that took this constant into account. Tom had become a lawyer. Christine had married one of the most promising junior partners in the firm. They couldn't help themselves; the firm was in their blood.

The only problem was that David had no ally when he wanted to play hooky from work. Not only would Chris not phone in sick for him, she couldn't comprehend why he would even consider doing such a thing. The firm was family business, and you didn't let your family down. David was lucky. The price tag for this loving marriage had not wedded him to an untenable professional situation. He was never called upon to do anything that made him relinquish the moral high ground. Bradhurst, Weiss, and Lowe was a first-class outfit. Some of the clients might be sleazebags, but their sleaziness was never allowed to tarnish the firm's reputation. Nor were the hours all that terribly demanding. Usually.

Still, David wished Christine wouldn't always be quite so understanding about the time he did put in on the job. A wife was supposed to be a little jealous of her husband's work-mistress. But Christine wasn't in the least, and sometimes David found that a little unnerving. How had he ended up with the perfect wife? They tell you to be careful what you wish for.

David sighed deeply, content with his fate. He was leading a charmed life. His was an existence thrice blessed, and he'd have to live with it.

He ruffled his wife's hair and asked, "Is Mr. Scarpelli going to be there?"

"I don't know. I didn't think to ask."

David grunted, feeling secretly vindicated, and turned his attention to wolfing down another forkful of scrambled eggs. At least she wasn't all-knowing.

∽∾∽∾∽

Traffic on I-75 was moderately heavy as David Vandemark sped along, heading for Detroit. His Olds 88 was running a little ragged. He made a mental note to take it into the shop for a tune-up this week. Being Motown born and bred, David reveled in the power of a big eight-cylinder engine. And why not? The Arab oil embargo was ancient history. The Japanese could keep their little pissant cars.

When David pulled up outside the Cass Avenue property, Horace Muldoon and Joseph Scarpelli were waiting for him. Scarpelli was a thin, bloodless little man who seldom showed any emotion. David always felt a bit uncomfortable around him and his cold, lifeless eyes. It was rumored that he had mob connections, but this had been said of every Italian businessman in Detroit at one time or another. David did put some credence in the stories he'd heard about Scarpelli, though. In the two years that the diminutive developer had been a client of the firm,

David had seen him push through half a dozen business deals with the lethal efficiency of a snake devouring a mouse. Everything about the man gave David the creeps.

No one in law school had ever said he would like all the people he'd have to take on as clients. Business was business, and a great deal of it was compromise. That was a part of the job David knew he could handle, provided he kept his contacts with Scarpelli to a minimum.

David couldn't help noticing that Muldoon, a contractor, appeared to defer to Joseph Scarpelli. Usually a loud and obnoxious bore, Muldoon was always on his best behavior around ol' Snake Eyes. He spoke deferentially to Scarpelli, even though he towered over the man by a good foot and a half and outweighed him by a hundred pounds. Muldoon's pungent, ever-present cigar was nowhere to be seen today, the definitive sign of respect.

﹢ For the next hour Muldoon and his monumental beer gut escorted his two companions around the silent, long-vacant tool and die plant. Their footsteps echoed through its cavernous depths. David and Scarpelli had both seen blueprints of what Muldoon's crew was supposed to do with the structure, but this was the first time they had actually been inside the building. David was appalled at how run-down it looked. Rain damage had decayed much of the top floor, and the seven floors below didn't look much better. From files he'd quickly skimmed that morning, David knew Scarpelli had hired another contractor to look at the property before he put down a nonrefundable binder. David was beginning to have his doubts about that other contractor's integrity and abilities. The building was in terrible shape.

Muldoon was echoing David's concern as he guided

them through the plant, but he assured Scarpelli there was nothing he couldn't fix. Only trouble was, it was going to cost a lot more money than anyone originally thought. Scarpelli greeted this news with a shrug and suggested that they retire to Muldoon's makeshift office on the ground floor to discuss the matter further.

As they waited for the ancient freight elevator to struggle up to the eighth floor, David looked around, trying to picture the place as the publishing offices of an as yet unborn magazine. That was what this floor was slated to become. He had seen this sort of metamorphosis occur many times, but he still couldn't help marveling at the ability of men like Muldoon to transform a dump like this into a modern and respectable place of commerce.

David's attention returned to his companions when he heard Scarpelli ask, "What about the elevators? Has that engineer been here yet?"

Muldoon responded good-naturedly, "Not yet, Mr. Scarpelli. Those college boys always got some lame excuse why they can't get the work done on time. This joker claims he's tied up with another job that's taking longer than he figured."

"Will this delay your getting started?"

"Afraid so, Mr. Scarpelli. Some of the equipment I'm going to have to bring up for the job is pretty heavy. I'm not sure these old clunkers can handle the load. Got to get them checked out first. Looks like they're fifty years old."

The sounds issuing from the elevator shaft made David surmise they probably hadn't been oiled in all that time. He considered suggesting they use the stairs to return to Muldoon's office, but decided against it at the last moment. He couldn't bring himself to show any sign of weakness or fear in front of Scarpelli. David silently cursed the man for eliciting such a male-dominance response in him. Lots of people didn't feel comfortable in elevators. It was nothing to be ashamed of. David put his misgivings aside, feeling rather silly about the whole thing.

After all, he'd been on elevators that sounded worse than this one. And none of them had ever broken down. Besides, Muldoon had probably inspected the elevator's power train and satisfied himself that the lift was safe enough to use in this kind of limited fashion. These elevators had been designed to carry several tons of freight. All three men combined couldn't weigh more than five hundred pounds.

When the elevator arrived, Muldoon slid open the wooden safety gate, then the inner doors of the freight compartment, and stepped inside the car. Scarpelli joined him, and both men turned questioningly toward David. He thought about claiming he'd dropped something and would meet them at the office, but he hesitated too long and Muldoon recognized the nervousness in his eyes.

"Come on, kid! It ain't gonna bite ya. I've been riding up and down in this rig all week. It's okay," he said, the invisible gauntlet of challenge lying on the floor between them. He waited beside the elevator's control panel for David's reply.

David noticed, with a mixture of embarrassment and relief, that the lift possessed the more modern push-button touch controls of new elevators. Incontrovertible proof that someone had worked on these elevators at least once in the last fifty years. He stepped into the cab with a slightly chagrined smile masking his irritation, aware of the powerful smell of decay. Damn that Muldoon for calling him out in front of a client.

Muldoon, obviously savoring the young lawyer's discomfort, pushed the lift doors shut and selected the ground floor. The elevator began its noisy descent. It traveled only one floor before coming to a jarring halt.

The lift then began lurching erratically up and down as a terrible cracking and rending noise came from above. David stepped nervously toward the back of the compartment, feeling helpless. No time now for recriminations. Muldoon stood transfixed, looking up toward the lift's unseen cables, gears, and engine. Scarpelli, displaying an unguessed-at agility, lunged for the elevator's control panel, shoving Muldoon out of the way.

"Move, you fat fool!" he screamed as he seized the elevator's emergency brake. The lift immediately ceased its frightening gyrations and the compartment filled with the sound of the elevator's distress siren.

Muldoon had lost his balance and fallen by the doors. He was trying to get to his feet and regain some of his lost dignity in the process. "Hell, Mr. Scarpelli, I was about to hit the brake myself. Ya didn't have to get tough about it."

Scarpelli ignored the fat man's admonitions. He and David were both listening intently to the continuing ominous sounds of grinding metal that could be heard above the wail of the distress siren. Some instinct told them what was about to happen and both men pressed themselves tightly against the wall of the car. Muldoon was trying vainly to convince Scarpelli that he was in control of the situation when the first section of the elevator's drive train came smashing through the car's ceiling.

It looked like some kind of support beam, but David couldn't be sure because he never got a good look at it. The beam crashed through the roof and buried itself in Muldoon. It pierced his right trapezius, continued into his chest cavity, and came to rest with only about nine inches of its three-foot length protruding. Muldoon stood there spurting blood, staring at Scarpelli and David, trying to say something. His lips moved, but nothing audible would ever pass through them again. Scarpelli and David watched this horrible parody of speech without attempting to guess what Muldoon wanted to say. David felt a tremendous desire to heave up his breakfast.

That sensation passed quickly, for mere seconds after the beam came through the ceiling the rest of the elevator's drive assembly followed, tearing through the enclosure. David's every muscle tightened instantly, bracing for death. The accumulated dirt and dust of fifty years rained down in a blinding cloud, making breathing difficult. As if by some suspension of the law of averages, none of the dozens of pieces of shrapnel struck either Scarpelli or David. Both men remained unhurt.

When David's vision cleared, he understood at once the gravity of their situation.

There were seven-foot holes in the roof and in the floor of the elevator. Two thick cables were racing each other down through the holes. Muldoon was nowhere in sight, the blood-splattered compartment mute testament to his recently departed presence.

Suddenly they heard something fly up past the elevator wall. What was that? No! Not the counterweight!

The counterweight slammed up into what was left of the elevator's rooftop drive assembly and jammed. David heard the sharp crack of cables snapping above him and threw himself into a corner. Scarpelli was rubbing the dirt from his eyes when the inch-thick cables, suddenly released from over 10,000 pounds of tension, came crashing through what was left of the elevator. Joseph Scarpelli saw the cable slice off his extended right hand and continue scything its destructive path down through the hole in the floor. He stared at his bloody stump as if wondering why it didn't hurt. Then a sudden wave of dizziness hit and he lost his balance, pitched head first into the void, silently plummeted down seven stories of darkness.

David heard Scarpelli's flight to eternity end with a sickening thud. He hadn't heard anything else hit bottom. Not the elevator's drive assembly, Muldoon, or the cables. He'd been too busy scrambling as deep into his corner of the elevator as he could manage. So far the effort had paid off. He was still alive. But for how long?

He surveyed his surroundings. Things didn't look good. What was left of the floor tilted toward the gaping hole in its center. Many of the seams in the elevator's walls were split and sitting at odd angles. What light there was filtered in through the hole in the ceiling from a skylight atop the elevator shaft. Everything inside the car was covered with blood. Even if he had someplace to go, moving around in this conveyance would be slippery and dangerous.

David decided to sit tight until help arrived. The distress siren had ceased blaring when the drive train crashed through the compartment, but surely someone on the street must have heard the terrible racket all this destruction and death had raised. Somebody would come to investigate or call for help. Then he remembered it was Saturday. Few people walked the streets of this warehouse district on weekends. He might be stuck here well into the night.

Christine would eventually call her father if David did not return home. Vincent Lowe would send someone to see if anything was wrong. Help would come sooner or later. All he had to do was remain calm and stay put. He would survive this nightmare somehow.

He huddled in the dim light wondering how Scarpelli and Muldoon had felt when they met their end. Had there been any last-minute flashes of understanding? Or had they checked out as scared and panic-stricken as David had felt witnessing their death? He knew he'd never know the answer to that. It's true, he thought grimly. Dead men tell no tales.

A cracking noise from above startled David so badly he nearly lost his grip on the waist-high handrail he'd been clinging to tenaciously. The crack was followed by a low grating sound. Good God, he thought, there can't be anything more left to fall, can there?

David knew there was only one way to find out. He pulled himself to his feet and took a few cautious steps toward the front of the elevator, never relinquishing his grip on the rail. When he reached the middle of the wall, he leaned out, looking up through the ragged hole in the ceiling.

There it was. It had to be the elevator's counterweight. Ripped loose from the rear wall, hanging precariously in the middle of the drive train's remaining support beams. How much did that thing weigh? At least half a ton, maybe more. When it fell, it would take out the rear section of the elevator, and David knew it couldn't hang there much longer. He moved cautiously toward the front of the elevator and the useless control panel.

Or was it useless? Wasn't there usually a phone behind the small rectangular door above the control panel? David edged closer and clawed at the panel until it opened.

The phone probably wouldn't have worked, even if the receiver hadn't been ripped out. David lowered himself to the floor, exhausted, resigned to his fate. He was back to waiting for someone to rescue him, only now he had to wonder whether they'd reach him in time.

As he thought about what had happened, David realized the elevator's emergency brake had held out incredibly well so far. Would it continue to do its job when the counterweight crashed into the cab? David doubted it. Either he would be rescued before the counterweight fell or he would die. It was as simple as that.

He closed his eyes and tried to remember a prayer from his childhood. His parents had never been religious. Neither was his aunt Ruth, with whom he later lived. In fact, the only prayers he'd ever learned were those that another aunt had taught him when he was five or six. He'd been able to recite five different "poems to God," as his aunt Shirley called them, before her two-week visit ended. But all of her efforts had been wasted. Now that he really needed them, he couldn't remember a single one.

A grating screech sounded overhead. It scraped across David's nerves as if they were violin strings. David tried to ignore it.

He let his mind wander, hoping to lose himself in reverie. His thoughts turned to his wife and child. What would Chris and Jenny do if he didn't make it? Would Christine remarry? Would Jenny eventually learn to call his replacement Daddy?

Those were stupid thoughts. David Vandemark was still among the living, and he was damn well going to stay that way. He wasn't sure how, but he would beat this situation. It didn't matter that the odds were incredibly long. Had it been only a few short hours ago that he'd been thinking about how charmed his life was? A charmed existence was not meant to end in such a squalid manner.

David's thoughts were punctuated by a terrible cracking noise. He squeezed his eyes shut and curled himself into a ball. He was only vaguely aware of the impact of the counterweight crashing through the compartment, followed by the unsettling sensation of falling. All he could grasp was the fear. It was like a rabid creature inside him. His eyes sprang open and an inhuman shriek of terror erupted from his throat. This agonized scream seemed to go on forever, filling the plummeting compartment, echoing up the elevator shaft. Just as it seemed that David's mind would shatter like glass from the intensity of that howl, his world exploded into all-encompassing pain. The banshee stopped howling. Then darkness fell, and silence came to rest once more.

8

July 14, 1996
War Memorial Park, Washington, D.C.

"Vandemark survived the crash, of course, but it was touch-and-go for a while." Ira paused in his narrative as he and Vida strolled past the somber black marble monolith of the Vietnam War Memorial. Tourists, most of whom passed by slowly, were quietly respectful of those who stopped to reverently touch the names inscribed there. "They actually lost him on the operating table at one point. His heart stopped, but they resuscitated him. Better they hadn't."

Vida, her curiosity piqued, asked, "Do you really think everyone might have been better off if they hadn't resuscitated him?"

"Absolutely. If Vandemark had checked out like he was supposed to, you and I wouldn't be working on this thankless assignment."

Vida was appalled by Ira's cynicism. "But Vandemark's victims would still be alive."

"Well, we wouldn't want that!"

"You make it sound as if Vandemark did everyone a favor by murdering . . . what did you say it was, eighteen people?"

"As far as we know. In some ways those killings did a lot of good. Damn lot of good. But let me lead up to that my own way, okay?"

"Your way is beginning to drive me nuts, Ira. For an hour you've been filling me in on this case, and I still don't know who Vandemark killed."

"I want you to understand what sort of strange bird we're after. First rule of the hunt: You have to know your prey before you can track him."

Vida threw her hands up in mock surrender. "All right. You're the boss."

Ira settled himself on a park bench facing the Vietnam Memorial. Vida, beside him, was experiencing a disorienting if not entirely unpleasant sense of unreality, as if she had stepped through a looking glass and Ira and the curious players of this story were the strange creatures beyond it.

"You know, Vida, Vandemark was in the National Guard. He was too young for Vietnam, but Uncle Sam spent a pile of money teaching him how to kill. Now the government pays us to bring him down for using that skill."

They sat without speaking for a few moments. Then Vida said, "You were going to tell me what happened in the hospital."

"David was in a coma for two weeks after the operation. He'd fractured his skull in the fall, broken his leg in two places, cracked a couple of ribs. It was only the head injury doctors worried about, though.

"Dr. Philip Craigmore, a neurosurgeon, performed the operation that relieved fluid buildup inside Vandemark's skull. Craigmore watched over him while he was comatose, even tried to help him after he regained consciousness, but Vandemark didn't do too well in rehabilitation. Guess he was pretty well gone by then."

"Gone?" Vida repeated. "Did he suffer brain damage?"

"That's what Craigmore thought at first. When Vandemark came to, it was like some wires had gotten crossed; he didn't talk, couldn't seem to understand what anyone was saying, spent his first forty-eight hours of consciousness hiding under the sheets, crying about 'too many voices.' Everyone thought he was suffering from complete auditory and verbal dysfunction. They decided something in his brain was busted, so maybe he could hear words but couldn't make sense of them. Craigmore told me some folks who have head injuries like Vandemark's wind up like stroke victims. That's what they thought they were dealing with in David's case."

"It wasn't?"

"No. Two days later David Vandemark started talking and understanding people just fine. His speech was a little slurred, like he'd been drinking, but otherwise he was okay. They never did find out what was upsetting him in the beginning. Vandemark said he had no memory of his first forty-eight hours."

"How was he after that?"

"Meshugas . . . crazy. Dr. Craigmore told me David couldn't get out of the hospital fast enough. During the time he was in a coma, they only had an air cast around his busted leg. When he came to, it was all they could do to keep him immobilized long enough to wrap the leg in plaster. No one in the hospital'd ever seen a patient recover faster from such serious injuries. He wouldn't even stick around for observation. David was determined to hit the road, and no one was going to stop him."

"What'd the accident do? Turn him into a superman?"

"Ah, now that's the question, isn't it? It certainly turned him into something strange. One of the reasons they didn't want him to leave the hospital was that something distinctly peculiar had happened to Vandemark during the time he was comatose. This became blatantly apparent when Craigmore had David's father-in-law, Vincent Lowe, break the bad news to Vandemark about his family. It was David's response to the tragedy that really floored them.

"When Lowe told him, as gently as possible, that his wife and child had been murdered while he was unconscious, he didn't blink an eye. No tears, no rage. He said he already knew, and in the same breath he began to pester Craigmore about getting discharged from the hospital."

"Someone on the staff told him?"

"That's what Craigmore concluded. He was furious and spent the next week acting like a Spanish inquisitor general. No one owned up to it. I interviewed most of the staff later on, and I don't think any of them told David about the murders."

"Then how do you think he found out?"

"I have no idea. That was the first of many strange occurrences connected with this case I would come across. The more I've learned about Vandemark over the last seven years, the less it seems I understand."

"They let him out of the hospital?"

"Yes, he was released into Vincent Lowe's care, but that didn't last long. Two days later, while her husband was at work, Mrs. Lowe went shopping for groceries. When she got back, the guest room was empty and there was a note on the bed. David had called a cab and taken off.

"Lowe went over to David's place that evening. He found his son-in-law sitting in his own living room, cleaning a thirty-eight semiautomatic. This worried Lowe. He thought David might be entertaining thoughts of suicide, but before he got a chance to voice this fear, David glibly assured him he'd bought the gun for protection.

"Turned out it was an example of the most striking new facet of David Vandemark's personality after the accident. I've talked to literally dozens of people who dealt with him during that time, and they all claim David developed an annoying habit of answering questions before they were asked. Strange, no?"

"Telepathy?"

"That's one theory. I think it has more to do with most people being pretty predictable."

Vida tried to sort through these bizarre details as Ira dug a cigar out of his coat pocket and lit it. Blue smoke billowed from his lips. "David became kind of a recluse at that point. Reportedly spent a lot of time in his basement, cut himself off from all his old friends, didn't seem to want them around anymore, didn't talk much. When he did go out, he was rude, antisocial. Even Vincent Lowe stopped coming around after one particularly disturbing incident. Vandemark eventually quit the firm, started living off his savings. Friends tried to get him to see a shrink, but he claimed it would simply be a waste of time."

Vida leaned forward, looking at the war memorial without seeing it. "I have no idea where you're heading with all this. I thought for a second you were about to tell me Vandemark killed his own family."

"That's what a few of the local police thought later on. Entertained the notion it was a contract killing that got messy. But that idea didn't wash. Vandemark loved his wife and child. I think it was their death that pushed him over the edge."

"If Vandemark didn't kill them, who did?"

"This animal I was after at the time. He'd done four women in the area and was virtually impossible to get a lead on. The Bureau got involved when he decided to raise the stakes by dumping the last body just over the state line. Four murders and not a single usable shred of forensic evidence. The Detroit police dubbed him Mr. Clean."

9

Greg Hewett backed his battered old Volkswagen into the parking space in front of the trailer. He was returning from the supermarket with a couple days' worth of food, a six-pack of Bud, and a copy of the *Detroit News*.

Stepping out of the car, he glanced up and down the deserted roads of the Southfield trailer park he called home. He hated the place. No one ever hung around outside, even on a warm afternoon like this. They were inside their little air-conditioned trailers, free from the heat and the possibility of being bothered by someone passing by. Greg missed the Memphis, Tennessee, suburb he'd grown up in. There was always someone sitting on a porch in Oakville, someone he could jaw with before going into his own house. Not here, though. These damn Yankees locked themselves into their little metal boxes like someone was after them. Well, maybe someone was.

It was a good place to hide out; that was why Greg Hewett had chosen to live in this crummy little trailer park. He'd been here almost a year and didn't know any of his neighbors by their first names. To them, he was

Hewett in unit 7 on Ford Road. The streets in this dump were named for cars. More of that Motor City jive.

Three years ago Greg had gone by the tag Gregory Walton, his real name. But then he'd gotten into trouble back in Oakville and had to change it whenever he moved. Which was about once a year. He never heard the baying of hounds or the tramp of pursuing feet exactly, but Greg knew they were still looking for him. After all, he had broken the ultimate taboo, and he continued to do so every time the hunger hit him. He realized they'd catch him someday, but he didn't care anymore. The only time he truly felt alive these days was when the hunger was upon him. He'd stopped trying to fight it long ago.

Once inside his trailer, Greg stored the groceries, popped open a Bud, and sat down to read the paper. There was nothing on the front page that interested him. Greg didn't give a shit what was happening on the national and international fronts. He got the paper to find out what was going on in Detroit. He figured Motown was his stomping ground for now, and it was best to know what was going down around you if you didn't want to get stomped.

Greg scanned the local news, mildly amused by what he found there. There was an article on Mayor Young. Hewett had been floored when he found out Detroit had a colored mayor, but he supposed it made sense: the town had more niggers than any place he'd ever lived. That was why he'd moved into this trailer park, far from the Sterling stamping plant where he worked. Sure, it was ratty, but at least it was still all white.

He continued flipping through the paper, but nothing caught his interest until he got to page ten. It was her picture that grabbed him. The photo was right next to an article about an elevator accident in downtown Detroit. There was a picture of some clown right beneath the photograph of her and this man walking through a parking lot. The old coot had his arm around her. That annoyed Greg. The creep looked ancient enough to be her father.

When he read the article and the captions, he discovered that the old creep was indeed her father and the bozo in the photo below was her lawyer husband. He'd survived that elevator accident and was laid up at Beaumont Hospital.

Greg Hewett stared intently at the blurry screened photo of Christine Vandemark being led through the hospital parking lot. There was something sexy about her sad and helpless look. He liked the way the morning sun made her hair shine. Was she a blonde? Probably. Greg liked blondes. They'd always been his favorites.

The article stated that the Vandemarks lived in Warren, but it didn't give an address. Greg got up and fetched the phone book. He sat down on the couch and looked up David Vandemark. There he was! Greg had been afraid a lawyer might have an unlisted number. Guess he ain't that successful yet, he thought.

Christine Vandemark. He liked the name. Sounded good when he said it out loud. With her husband in the hospital she'd be all alone and frightened; she'd need comforting. Greg was very good at comforting.

It had been a couple months since he had let the hunger have its way. He'd been watching the papers; there'd been no mention of his little adventures being linked together yet. He'd traveled some each time he quenched the hunger. One time he'd gone as far as Ohio.

Greg made a point of not doing his thing in the same county twice. He felt reasonably safe. There was no need to disappear until the local cops spotted the pattern. He'd been very careful in Michigan. Careful about choosing his partners. Careful in comforting them.

Greg pushed himself up off the couch and headed for the bathroom, savoring the warm, tight feeling he had inside his well-worn jeans. On the way, he flipped on the radio. Hendrix's "All along the Watchtower" filled the air. He stripped at the bathroom door, tossing his clothes onto the hall rug. Then he grabbed a can of shaving cream and began to shake it up to the rhythm of the music.

He stepped into the bathtub and began to lather up slowly, enjoying the feel of the menthol cream against his skin. The music began working its magic, and he started to hum along as he switched blades on the razor. Greg reminded himself not to bounce to the beat. He didn't want to cut himself when he was about to go visiting. Take it slow and easy. Make a clean job of it. He started on his left foot and worked his way up the leg.

10

Ira Levitt could never stomach murder. The only thing he liked less was visiting the scene of the crime. In his twenty-one years with the Bureau, Ira had been at only two murder scenes, and both had made him violently ill. He could handle photos and forensic evidence that other agents collected. That material was removed enough from reality. But surveying the actual premises, seeing firsthand the cruelty one human could inflict upon another, was more than Ira could handle, and yet he got assigned to more than his share of homicides. Maybe because he had proved himself such an excellent tracker of killers. His revulsion probably spurred him on, gave him the edge he needed to crack these cases.

Ira usually found an excuse to stay away from the crime scene until the bodies had been removed and the blood had had a chance to dry, but he wasn't so lucky today. He'd been going over some files down at Detroit Police headquarters when the call came in: Mr. Clean had struck again, this time in the suburb of Warren. Bryan Cruz, the Detroit homicide detective assigned to the Mr. Clean case, had offered to give Ira a lift, and Ira, caught off guard and wishing he could develop a sudden appendicitis attack or minor brain seizure, found himself heading for the site of Mr. Clean's latest massacre.

Mr. Clean was a messy worker, even if he did straighten up afterward. Ira thanked heaven that he had decided to skip lunch and that Cruz hadn't wanted to talk about the case on the drive up. Most of the way, the Detroit cop had rambled on about a recent trip to Utah. It had helped keep Ira's mind off what lay ahead.

He felt a great sense of relief when he saw two attendants carrying a body bag toward a waiting ambulance as Cruz parked the car.

Cruz was furious. "Damn! They were supposed to wait until we got here!"

Ira looked down the quiet suburban street at the seemingly endless rows of brick and aluminum-sided houses with their carefully kept lawns. It was hard to believe anything as sordid as murder could take place in such a setting. But half a dozen years on the job had taught him that even nice people got killed occasionally. It seemed surreal every time he pulled such a case.

Bryan was bitching about the bodies as they got out of the car. Levitt tried to sound conciliatory. "Guess the word didn't get to them in time. Looks like we'll have to satisfy ourselves with what your forensic team digs up."

"I want to get a feel for the scene. Let's check it out."

Ira reluctantly followed the detective into the house. His stomach had been revolting on him for the last half hour. It was beginning to settle down now that the prospect of viewing the butchered remains of some poor woman had faded. He could handle inspecting the house.

Then a uniformed attendant passed him in the doorway. He was gently carrying a half-filled body bag out to the ambulance. Dear God, no . . . a child. Levitt's stomach did a backflip. He felt around in his pockets for the roll of Tums he habitually carried.

Ira popped one in his mouth as he noticed a portrait hanging on the wall of the living room. The three people in the photo had to be the family who lived here: husband, wife, and daughter. The woman and child had golden blond hair. The man's was light brown. They looked happy. Ira turned away. He had seen enough.

By that time, Cruz had talked to one of the officers on duty and was signaling Ira to follow him downstairs. Same M.O. Practically all they had to go on with Clean. Each of Clean's alleged murders had taken place in the basement of the victim's own home, though the fourth woman had later been discovered in a wooded area across the state line.

The floor of this basement was tiled. Imitation wood paneling covered the walls, and there was an acoustical-tile ceiling. Toys littered the floor and spilled from the wooden chest in one corner. Nearby sat a rather worn sofa, probably the predecessor of the couch up in the living room. On the other side of the room, a washer and dryer stood beside a sorting table and sink. The garden hose was ominously connected to the faucet. Most of the hose lay coiled neatly on the wet floor.

This was Mr. Clean's work, all right. Not a spot of blood to be seen anywhere; everything had been carefully hosed down. Levitt could see that the tape used to mark the position of a homicide victim had proved useless on the damp floor. A large wadded-up ball of it lay on the sorting table. Someone had outlined the position of the corpses in Magic Marker instead.

Warren police had requested the loan of Detroit's forensic team. They were busily at work, so Cruz and Levitt remained by the stairs, observing the proceedings. One detective was shooting pictures of the scene. Another was dusting for prints in the drier sections of the basement. A third was down on his hands and knees beside a drain in the center of the floor. He had the grill off and was scraping sludge from the rim with a penknife, then transferring the mess to an evidence bag.

A fourth man, tall and balding, came over to Cruz and Levitt. Bryan introduced him. "Ira Levitt, FBI. This is George Schuster, coroner's office. What you got, George? This Clean's work?"

"Who else? How many homicidal maniacs tidy up after themselves? Our boy's been at it again, no doubt about it."

Cruz looked around. "Same routine. Anything new this time?"

"Only the little girl. This is the first time we know of that he's whacked a kid," said Schuster.

"Rape her too?"

"We'll have to get confirmation from the lab, but my guess is that he just beat her head in with a blunt object, probably his gun. Our boy may be a lot of things, but he's no pedophile. I figure he killed the kid because she was in his way."

"How'd it go down?"

"About the same as the first four. No signs of forced entry. Either the lady let him in or he came in through an unlocked entrance, probably the front door. It looks like it's been wiped down.

"Once inside, Clean herded them into the basement.

My guess is that's when he strips down and pulls out the knife and rubber gloves. The woman had a pretty good-sized lump on her head. So, considering the amount of swelling, she was alive for quite a while after he hit her. Clean probably tapped her one, to get her out of his hair while he pistol-whipped the child. Then he waited for her to come around, so he could have his fun with her.

"Raped and sodomized her, then cut her up. Lots of mutilation around the breasts, buttocks, and vaginal area. Never touches their faces, though. That's one of Clean's odd quirks. These loonies usually like to slash up the area around the mouth."

"Then he cleaned the place up, just like always, huh?"

"Yeah, he used the garden hose from the backyard; you can still see the impression in the grass. Rinsed the basement down and went on his merry little way. He would have had to get dressed to go out and get the hose. We're checking with the neighbors to see if anyone spotted him then or when he arrived or left."

A sour expression drifted across Cruz's features. "Don't hold your breath. I'm beginning to think this guy's invisible. No one ever sees him coming or going. He's now murdered six people in the Detroit area, and we haven't got the slightest idea what he looks like."

"That's because the sneaky son of a bitch knows something about forensics. I tell you, this guy doesn't leave a scrap of physical evidence. No way for us to get a mental picture of him. He even uses condoms when he rapes his victims. You ever hear of anything like that? There's no semen left to get a blood type."

"How do you know he's not just shooting blanks?" Ira asked.

George Schuster looked at Ira. "You new on this case?"

"Yeah, I was brought in when Clean dropped that body over the state line into Ohio. It became federal then. Kidnapping and transporting. You know the drill."

"Okay, when you get to the file on Mrs. Jane Rice, the woman he did in Hamtramck, you'll see that we found a condom wrapper left behind at the scene. No prints. No used rubber. He must take them with him. I think he left the wrapper on purpose. These types like to show the cops how clever they are. That's what generally trips them up in the end."

Cruz stepped closer to the larger of the two outlined forms on the floor and bent down, trying to visualize the missing body. "He scrape everything out from under her nails?"

"A manicurist couldn't have done a better job. This guy isn't a biter, either. No teeth impressions. No way we'll ever be able to identify him by his choppers or dental records. No fingerprints. No telltale pubic hairs left behind. I'm willing to bet this creep shaves every inch of himself before he makes a hit. That's the only logical way he wouldn't leave some type of fiber evidence behind."

Abruptly Ira asked, "What do you make of his knowing so much about forensics?"

"Who knows? Maybe he read a book. Maybe he is or was a cop. God, I hope not. There's half a dozen other ways I can think of how he could have picked up the know-how. I don't expect you'll get anywhere along that track."

Cruz stood up and walked back over to Ira and the coroner. "You never can tell. There was this dude slashing prostitutes downtown. At first we thought he was just picking his victims at random. But it turned out they all went to the same place to get their hair done. Took us a while to tumble to this because we thought the only common factor among the victims was that they were all hookers. Then one day this beautician calls up to tell us they were all customers of hers at one time or another. Turned out the beautician's husband was the killer. He didn't like his wife associating with lowlifes."

"Yeah, I guess you can never tell." George turned to give the photographer some instructions.

Cruz nudged Levitt and headed for the stairs. "C'mon. Nothing more to see here. Let's go get some dinner. They won't have the preliminary autopsy and forensic reports ready for at least another three hours."

Ira Levitt wasn't crazy about the idea of food at that moment, but he was relieved to get out of the basement. There hadn't been any blood or bodies, true, but the place reeked of carnage. It wasn't a smell exactly, but Ira could feel the effluvium of death on his bare skin, taste it in the air. He wanted out of there, and fast. His stomach was turning to pure acid.

Once upstairs, Cruz stopped to talk to a uniformed officer in the kitchen. Levitt walked toward the front of the house, stopping by the foyer. He glanced at the photo of the family again. The woman smiled at him.

"Raped and sodomized her, then cut her up. Lots of mutilation around the breasts, buttocks, and vaginal area."

Levitt felt his gorge rise. He bolted through the front door, raced around the corner out of sight, and threw up over a sewer grating.

He'd recovered his composure and straightened up by

the time the other officer came out of the house. As Cruz pulled his car away from the curb, heading for a chop suey joint on Fourteen Mile Road, Ira swore this was absolutely the last time. No more murders. He'd quit the Bureau before he let them assign him to another murder case.

11

Ira examined his spent stogie, dropped it to the sidewalk, and extinguished it with his formidable shoe. "What happened to Vandemark's family was enough to send anyone around the bend. Add to that the elevator accident and the guy never had a chance of getting his shit together again."

"Let me see if I have this right," said Vida. "You're saying Vandemark had no part in any plot to kill his wife and child."

"That's what I'm saying. But it's just my read of the facts. Bryan Cruz would probably debate the point. He thinks Vandemark and Clean had some kind of deal going. His argument: how else would David know where to find Clean?"

"Sounds like a key question."

"That and something Vincent Lowe told Cruz later on convinced Bryan that Vandemark was involved in the murder of his wife and kid."

"The 'one particularly disturbing incident' you mentioned earlier?"

"Right the first time. Give the lady a cigar."

"No, thanks."

"Lowe stopped by Vandemark's place unexpectedly after work one night. No one answered the door, but Lowe was sure David had to be home. He got worried and let himself in."

"And found what, exactly?"

"David buck-ass naked, except for the leg cast, crawling around on that Magic Marker outline on the basement floor."

"Where his wife's body was found?"

"Yeah. Lowe claimed Vandemark was in a stupor. The old guy had a hell of a time dragging his son-in-law upstairs and cleaning him up. Apparently Vandemark pissed himself."

"Total regression. Could be . . ." said Vida mostly to herself, fascinated by the notion of fugue and other altered states of being.

"Cruz is convinced it was a perverse sex ritual—that Vandemark was screwing his dead wife."

"You buy that?"

"No. Whatever Vandemark was doing is still a mystery, far as I'm concerned. But it must have acted as some kind of catalyst. The very next day things really escalated."

12

Something had disturbed Laura Menguelli's sleep. She thought perhaps it had been a sound, only half heard through layers of deep slumber. Now as she lay in bed, alert and a little frightened, she wondered if the noise might have been part of a forgotten dream. The first-floor flat she shared with her parents and kid brother on Ninety-seventh Street in Elmhurst was quiet and still. Laura's eyes sought the luminous face of her alarm clock: 3:18 A.M.

Laura lay there, trying to regulate her breathing, hoping that would let her drift back to sleep. After all, there was nothing to be afraid of, and she needed to catch some z's. That math exam first thing in the morning would be tough enough without having to tackle it half asleep.

Thinking of school made her realize why she was so on edge. It was all Billy Sherman's fault. Yesterday during lunch break, that geek had started going on and on about those killings that had been in the papers lately: the ones *El Diario* called the Latino Family Murders.

Laura shivered at the memory. Sherman had gleefully described in graphic detail the condition in which the last family had been found: slashed, mutilated. They were the fourth family slaughtered in such a manner in the last two months. Someone had crept into their house in the middle of the night, killed them, and then dismembered them. The neighbors had heard nothing. And no one had survived any of these gruesome attacks to give the police any leads. The only common thread, it seemed, was that the victims all had Hispanic surnames.

Billy Sherman had gotten a real kick out of telling Laura that the Slasher was going to get her and her family. He suggested they get busy changing their name to Smith or Jones. "Hey Laura, what's Spanish for 'bogeyman'?" he'd joked. What an asshole!

Annoyed with herself for having let that nerd get to her, Laura squeezed her eyes shut, trying to will herself back to sleep. It didn't work. That was the trouble with having a keen mind: it usually came equipped with an overactive imagination. Laura sighed and stared up at the ceiling. Maybe a glass of milk would help.

She got up and made her way to the kitchen without turning on a light. The glare inside the refrigerator was blinding, so she decided to enjoy her late-night drink in the dark; lights would only make it harder to fall asleep afterward. Damn that Billy Sherman. The only reason she even talked to the jerk was because of his pal, Sergio Funaro. Sergio was a new face at school, a transfer from some Catholic high school in Brooklyn. Sitting in the dark thinking of Sergio gave Laura a warm feeling. She remembered turning around and catching Sergio staring at her the other day. It wasn't the first time she'd caught him. She thought it was kind of cute. Laura liked the way he looked at her. Sergio was a year older, a senior, but that only made him more of a challenge. Laura smiled at the thought of rising to it.

A door opened and closed, so quietly that Laura almost missed it. The sound had come from one of the bedrooms down the hall. She waited patiently, but no one joined her in the kitchen. A moment later she heard another door open and close. This door creaked a little. That was how she knew it was José's room. Her brother was probably returning from a late-night call of nature.

José. Laura had been worrying about her brother lately. He'd been acting strangely. José was two years younger, at that age where mood changes could signify one of two things: the onset of puberty, or drug abuse. Laura prayed it wasn't the latter. As far as she was concerned, drugs were just a slow form of suicide. She'd lost a good friend last year to a cerebral hemorrhage while smoking crack. Sixteen years old and dead. Please, dear God, let it be puberty with José. *That* you eventually get over.

She remembered her own bout with blossoming womanhood. For a while her own mood changes had almost made her crazy. Thank God she'd gotten past that stage. At the ripe old age of seventeen, Laura felt that the worst was behind her.

But what about José? Was it budding sexuality or dope? It seemed to Laura that more than half the kids at Roosevelt High were frying their brains on coke, crack, or heroin. She thought José had enough sense to avoid that trap, and she hoped her own example had helped him learn to say no, but you can never be sure. "Laura, you're beginning to sound like an anti-drug commercial," José had said.

Then Laura heard another noise from the back of the house. This time it didn't sound like a door. More like a moan or cry. Someone having a dream? Before she could make up her mind, the creak of José's door sounded again, followed by dead silence.

Leaving her glass of milk half finished, Laura got up and looked into the hallway leading to the three bedrooms, having grown accustomed to the dark by now. No one was in the hall. The doors to both José's room and her own stood ajar. Laura tried to remember whether she'd closed hers on the way out, but she couldn't recall.

She walked to José's door and peered inside, but she couldn't make out her brother. A streetlight provided some illumination, but most of the bed was a shadow. "José?" she whispered tentatively. No response. "José?" A little louder this time. Still nothing. He must be really out of it, she decided.

As Laura took a step toward her own room, the milk forgotten, she stepped in something wet and sticky with her bare foot. In the dim light, it looked like ink. Then came a dreadful realization. "Mother of God!" A quick intake of breath and a whispered, "José!"

The light switch was at the end of the hall. Laura stumbled toward it, suddenly terrified, no longer sure of her footing. She flipped the switch and was immediately blinded by the glare of two naked 75-watt lightbulbs. A second later her eyesight cleared, and there it was, on the hallway floor, just as she'd feared. Blood.

Drops and smears of blood on the floor and walls.

"José?"

Laura could barely force herself to return to the doorway of her brother's room, terrified by the prospect of what she might find. All she could see was the foot of José's bed. She pushed the door open farther. As she did so, the illumination from the hall light silently crept up the length of the bed. Only when the door was wide open could Laura see her brother's face. His eyes were open, staring at . . . nothing. His mouth was open too. A small trickle of scarlet ran from the corner of his lips, across his cheek and into his hair. But that wasn't the only blood. The sheets beneath his chin were soaked in it. Blood! Blood everywhere!

"Oh my God! Oh, God! Jesus, no! Popeeeee!"

Laura whirled and raced to the end of the hall, to her parents' room. She yanked open the door, screaming, "Popi! Mami! It's José! He's hurt himself! He's . . . he's . . ."

Her father's eyes were wide open, glassy. Her mother stirred not at all, her eyes closed, sleeping peacefully. She would sleep like this forever. The floral-patterned sheets were streaked and splattered with bloody flowers, bright crimson in the harsh glare of the hallway light. Laura stood there, her jaws moving but no sound coming out. She could feel tears beginning to run down her cheeks.

Then the lights went out behind her. Some part of her howled, begging Laura to run. But her body refused to obey. Frozen. Scream, dammit! she told herself, but that too proved impossible. The sound of muffled footsteps came toward her. Someone grabbed her hair and pulled her head back. Laura felt something brush against her throat, then a wetness on her chin and collarbone.

She finally worked up the courage to scream, but it was too late. All that came out was a wretched gurgling noise. She touched her neck, felt the wet stickiness, then the slit. The world dropped out from under her. She felt herself falling. Laura was vaguely aware of her body twitching on the floor, like that spasm as you fall asleep, just before all sensation ceased. Forever.

13

The digital readout on his watch said 5:47 A.M. Charles Camden looked through the window of his chauffeur-driven limousine at the street people haunting Times Square. He was not surprised to see them at this hour. They were here every morning as the sun rose behind the skyscrapers.

The limo turned right on Forty-second Street and glided past all-night porno theaters and peep shows, rolling along until it reached the far west side of Manhattan, then turned downtown and continued. It came to a stop outside a warehouse on a pier. Camden assessed the exterior of the dilapidated building, satisfied that anyone driving by would surely wonder why this old fossil hadn't been torn down decades ago. It was the perfect cover, blended in seamlessly with the rest of this decaying area; a neighborhood waiting for salvation in the form of major renovation that might never come.

That impression remained when Camden stepped into the warehouse's front office. An unshaven, cigar-smoking blimp of a man watched him through little piggy eyes from behind a chain-link partition, acknowledging Camden's arrival with a curt nod. Camden noticed the peeling paint in the office, the garbage-strewn floor. Yes, it certainly was perfect. Perfectly disgusting. Anyone walking in off the street would want to go no further.

A closed-circuit video camera relayed Camden's image to a computer bank, where it was identified and cataloged. The computer returned a clearance signal, and a buzzer sounded, unlocking the door in front of him. Camden pushed it open and stepped through. The blimp behind the partition flipped the safety back on his Uzi and put the weapon back in its usual place, an otherwise empty file drawer labeled U. A private joke.

Camden inspected his image in the full-length mirror inside the door. He knew it was two-way, with an armed guard behind it, but it served his purpose nonetheless. Camden smoothed his jacket and straightened his tie, ran a hand through his thick graying hair. At fifty-nine, Charles Camden was every bit as meticulous about his image and appearance as he had been at twenty. He looked like the high-power executive he was; there was raw power in his carriage and manner. Nothing in his thirty years of service had diminished the fire in his eyes. Power agreed with him. His sharp gray eyes gleamed with satisfaction at the figure he saw in the mirror. He gave himself a wink and moved on.

Camden marched down the freshly painted pea-green hallway to his office. He opened the unmarked oak door, stepped in, and found two men sitting on a sofa in the reception area. Camden stepped through to his private section without a word. A slight tilt of his head was the only indication to the two men that he wanted them to follow. Both of them maintained a stony silence until Camden had sat down behind his large mahogany desk and said, "Well?"

The taller of the two men—slim, with a dark brown crew cut and glasses—said, "Hanson and McGuire called in. The operation went off without a hitch, sir."

As Camden turned in his chair, his eyes gravitated to the imposing Gainsborough landscape hanging on the wall behind his desk. "How were the telemetry and biofeedback readings?"

The other man, heavier and redheaded with a bushy mustache, nervously cleared his throat. "Exactly as expected, sir. Would you like me to send up a detailed read-out?"

Lost in thought within the landscape, Camden replied slowly, deliberately, "No, that won't be necessary. Just give me a run-through of the highlights."

Looking perplexed by this request, the redhead glanced at his companion for support or advice, found neither, shrugged his shoulders, and began to read off number codes and time-frame references from the sheaf of papers he held.

Camden listened to the man's litany for maybe three seconds before the crisply pronounced numbers faded from his consciousness. Though he continued to gaze at the Gainsborough, that too faded for him. In its place lay the slashed and murdered bodies of Hernando and Maria Menguelli and their children, José and Laura. A smile spread across Camden's face. It lingered until the red-headed man finished his recital and asked if there'd be anything else.

14

Vida, working on her second cup of coffee, impatiently checked her watch for the umpteenth time. She was supposed to have met Ira for breakfast twenty minutes ago. Apparently punctuality wasn't one of her new partner's virtues. But Vida wasn't going to hold that against him. Ira was perhaps the first person in the Bureau who hadn't treated her like either an affirmative action annoyance or a sex object. That absolved him of a multitude of sins.

Besides, Vida nearly hadn't made it out of bed this morning herself. The temptation to turn off the alarm and roll over for another six or eight hours of sleep had been almost overwhelming. She had stayed up reading the David Vandemark files until nearly two-thirty. Fascinating reading. Almost unbelievable, in fact. But that wasn't what made getting up this morning so difficult. Mom had called from Baltimore earlier in the evening.

Vida wondered why mother-daughter relationships were so difficult. Mom meant well, and Vida believed that her main purpose in calling was to make certain her little girl had settled comfortably in Washington. But five minutes into their conversation, when Vida thought it was safe to relax, her mother had reminded her yet again how much was riding on her doing well at the Bureau and graduating from law school.

Vida's father, Malcolm Johnson, had been Baltimore's most successful black lawyer. At least that was what everybody had thought. He'd had prestigious offices in the financial district, and his clients were some of the city's biggest corporations.

But Malcolm Johnson had run a one-man show. No senior partners, only a small army of associates. So at age fifty-two, hypertension having rendered the walls of his heart as thin as tissue paper, he succumbed to the inevitable heart attack. And the house of cards that was Malcolm Johnson and Associates collapsed. It turned out that he had taken a beating on a stock venture six months before his death. He hadn't told anyone in the family, figuring he could recoup his losses with eighteen months of hard work. But that wasn't to be. His secretary found him slumped over his desk one morning.

The insurance money had paid off the mortgage on the family home and allowed Vida to finish her last semester at college. Her mother had gotten a job as a legal secretary, which brought in enough to feed and clothe the family but not nearly enough for law school. Fortunately—or unfortunately, depending on how one looked at these things—an FBI recruiter had visited the college campus soon after Vida got the news about her family's financial situation. At the time it had seemed like an ideal trade-off: Vida got an opportunity to work within the legal system—not in the branch she was most interested in but in a job that would do for the present—and the

Bureau got a black female to help balance the racial equation that the politicians were forcing on it.

• There was an unspoken understanding in the family that once Vida passed the bar she would help put her three younger brothers through college. Vida knew it was a fair request. The only trouble was that dear well-intentioned Mom never let an opportunity pass to remind Vida how the entire family was depending on her. The three boys would surely turn to dope and become gangsters, she would say, if Vida screwed up on the job and blew their chance for a brighter future. Little wonder sleep always proved so elusive after a call from home.

Vida's reverie was interrupted when a meaty hand clapped her on the shoulder, making her jump.

"Steady there, lady. The vision may be ghastly but its intent is friendly," Ira said as he lowered himself onto the counter stool beside hers.

The vision was indeed ghastly: bloodshot and unshaven. Vida couldn't help staring with more than a little concern at her associate. "What happened to you?" she said at last.

After asking the waitress for a Danish and a cup of coffee, Ira said, "Ran into a couple of old friends on my way out of the office last night. We worked together on a murder case four years back. The three of us went off to a bar, started telling war stories. Before we knew it, it was two in the morning and we were plastered. Sorry I'm late."

"It's all right. I hope you enjoyed yourself last night. Looks like you're paying for it this morning. Did you work with those guys on the Vandemark case?"

"No, it was another murder case in Kentucky. The Bureau farms me out on odd jobs every so often. I've got a reputation for tracking killers, so they call me in on some of the tougher ones. 'Course, I always get transferred back to the Vandemark case before any arrests come down."

"That stinks."

"No, actually, it sucks. You get a chance to go through the file on Vandemark last night?"

The waitress arrived with Ira's coffee and Danish, and Vida watched him attack the food. "From beginning to end," she said. "It's amazing. There're parts I find hard to believe." She grimaced. "Aren't you going to feed your hangover anything better than that? Why not try something with a little protein?"

"Don't be a Jewish mother, Vida. Mine's still living, knock wood. But you're right, of course, about the Vandemark file and its air of unreality."

"There are some big gaps in his story right after he left the hospital."

Ira looked into his coffee cup, like a Gypsy reading tea leaves. "No one was paying much attention to him at the time. We all thought Vandemark was a grief-stricken wacko. Because of his fractured skull, he was regarded as a head case. Let's go. I'll tell you more about it on the way to the office."

The waitress brought Ira the bill and coffee to go, another Levitt tradition. Back on the street, Ira didn't seem eager to rush into his story, so Vida asked for some personal time off that morning, before he ruined his disposition by dredging up painful memories.

"Sure," he said. "Take the morning off. Nothing for you to do on the case today anyway. I want to run a few things through the major-cases computer upstairs. After that, we may have a trip to take."

"Really? Where?"

"Someplace where there's a lot of killing going on. I'll explain after lunch. Meet me at the Vietnam War Memorial at one-thirty."

They walked along in silence for a while. Vida sensed Ira was still priming himself to talk about Detroit in 1989. When the pair rounded a corner and the Federal Building came into view, Ira cleared his throat. "I never bought into the theory that Vandemark and Hewett worked together and later had a falling out. It just didn't wash in either direction. Hewett was a psycho loner. He and Vandemark would never have connected, wouldn't have had the opportunity."

"Then how do you explain it?"

"I can't, any more than I can explain the others. Vandemark seems to have a real rapport with the serial killer type. Maybe it's the 'it takes one to know one' principle at work. Anyway, I'd give an arm and a leg to know how he pulls it off."

Waiting for a traffic light to change, Vida said somewhat facetiously, "Maybe he consults a Ouija board, reads chicken guts, or does some other hoodoo shit."

"As good a guess as any. Maybe he came across a snitch the police missed. Maybe he has psychic dreams. He's beaten me to more serial murderers than I care to remember. Hell, he's got a better track record hunting these animals than the whole damn Bureau. All I know for sure is that when we went through Hewett's place a week later, we found all the evidence needed to convince ourselves that he was Mr. Clean. But by then it was too late."

15

Greg Hewett watched through a gap in the curtains. He didn't like what he saw. A black van had pulled up in front of his trailer, double-parking next to Hewett's car and blocking him in. Hewett had been packing, ready to move on to safer pastures. There'd been too many stories in the papers about the Mr. Clean killings. Time to hit the road. Time to say adios to Motown. The arrival of the van didn't bode well.

Greg pulled a .38 police special from a drawer without taking his eyes off the van. No one got out. Shit! Probably waiting for backup. That's how they would have done it back in Oakville when he was on the sheriff's department payroll.

Before Hewett could fan the flames of his paranoia any higher, the driver's door opened and a man stepped out. Greg felt himself relax. The driver appeared to be alone, and he didn't look like a cop. He was too well dressed: snappy sport coat, expensive-looking loafers. Cops didn't wear loafers, which could come off during a chase.

The man was carrying a brown folder. He looked around as if he wasn't quite sure where he was going.

Then he got a fix on Hewett's trailer and began limping toward it. That settled it; even this town wasn't hard up enough to use a gimpy cop. Greg had no way of knowing the man had sawed a fifteen-pound plaster cast off his leg less than two hours ago. He decided this character was going to try to sell him insurance or something. Greg would tell him to get lost and then get the hell out of here before anyone else showed up.

There was the expected knock on the door. Greg hid the gun under a magazine on top of the TV. The guy didn't look like a pig, but why take chances? There was something familiar about this character. Greg wondered if he'd seen him somewhere before.

Hewett opened the door and faced the stranger through the screen. Yeah, he definitely looked familiar. "Whatever you're selling, dude, I ain't interested."

The man outside the door smiled up at Greg. "Not selling anything," he said. "I'm here to give you something."

Having fended off more than one salesman since his arrival at the trailer park, Greg immediately put on his fiercest scowl and began to shut the door. "Can't afford it. Bye."

"I'm not a salesman. I'm a lawyer."

Lawyer? Hewett slowly opened the door a crack. The man was still standing there smiling, looking as if he knew something Greg didn't. Wary, Greg looked past the stranger. There were no cop cars quietly drifting into position. Nobody at all. Maybe this guy was legit. Maybe some kind of inheritance? No. Nobody knew who he was around here. Maybe something to do with the rent on the trailer. Could even be good news.

Deciding guessing games were a waste of energy, Greg

said, "What's this all about? I haven't got time to waste on bullshit."

The lawyer held up the brown folder and said, "If you're in a hurry, it'd probably be best if I gave you this so you can read it at your leisure."

Opening the screen door, Hewett asked, "What the fuck's this? Better not be anything you want to sell me."

"Take a look inside."

Greg took the folder and opened it. He was surprised to find only one typewritten sheet inside. Hewett was even more surprised when he read what the sheet said. So surprised, in fact, that he read it a second time before looking up at the stranger. By then the stranger had a gleaming black .38 automatic leveled at him.

Hewett looked back at the folder, trying to understand. He read the typed words one more time: "My name used to be David Vandemark. You murdered my wife and child. I want you to know who I am before I kill you."

So that was where he'd seen this guy before—in the paper. Greg flung the folder at the man's head and dived for the gun atop the television. His hand was closing around its grip when the first bullet ripped into his chest. Greg rocked back a couple of steps but kept his hold on the pistol. He was bringing it up when the second bullet hit him.

Greg Hewett sprawled on the floor like a bug on its back, feeling the life begin to drain out of him. He lifted his head and saw the two spreading scarlet pools on his shirt. He knew he was finished, could feel the blood filling his lungs, making it impossible to breathe. Greg turned toward the door. Through it, he could see the stranger calmly holstering the .38 under his sport coat.

He was certainly being cool about it. No fuss. No hurry. Very professional.

Hewett let his head fall back onto the floor. Lying there, looking up at the acoustical tiles on the ceiling, he began to laugh giddily.

∽∾∾∽

David Vandemark stood outside the trailer, listening to the shrill, girlish giggling. Hacking coughs eventually replaced the sound. He thought he heard the word "mother" between two coughing spasms, but he couldn't be sure. Finally all sound abruptly stopped. The silence was chilling.

He fished around in his coat pocket, pulled out several credit cards and other identification, and tossed them by the door of the trailer. Good-bye, Dave, ol' sport. There was already a new set of IDs in his wallet. David Vandemark, attorney-at-law, was dead; long live Charles Quinn, insurance adjuster. He had picked up the false driver's license, credit cards, and other bits of identification earlier in the week from a man David Vandemark had once defended on an assault charge. Hey, what were old friends for?

The past two weeks had been hectic. David had been busy selling his house at a great loss, liquidating his other assets and converting them to cash. The Oldsmobile had been traded in for a Ford Econoline, which he loaded with everything he thought he might need in his new life, which wasn't much—just some weapons and a few changes of clothing.

David Vandemark, a.k.a. Charles Quinn, limped to the

van. He checked to see if any of the neighbors had come out to see what all the shooting was about. No one had. Apparently no one cared that Greg Hewett had breathed his last, or that Mr. Clean had been fed his .38 caliber just desserts. They would read about it in the morning paper.

Charles Quinn climbed into the driver's seat of the van and found himself smiling at such thoughts. Thoughts that had been someone else's only moments ago.

It was time to hit the road. Time to say adios to Motown.

16

He was home. All it had taken was a cab ride from Penn Station to the bus terminal, then a Trailways bus to Woodstock, New York. He'd used his thumb the rest of the way. Once inside his quiet woodland cabin, he shed his Willard MacDonald identity and slipped into the persona the locals were used to: Vic Tanner, actor. His guise as a dinner theater thespian conveniently explained his long absences and his different hair colors. His reclusiveness was another aspect of the actor's temperament. No one from around those parts had set foot inside the old Butler place since Vic Tanner had taken possession. They would have been surprised at the changes in the old backwoods cabin.

Vic dropped his suitcases on the cot at the far end of the cabin's single room and looked around. Nothing had been disturbed. He found the nearly invisible hairs still wedged into the corners of his eight file drawers. The telltale hair between the shift and return keys on the computer was also where he had placed it. There'd been no break-ins, no snooping. The sanctity of his private domain had been preserved.

He walked to the kitchenette, opened the fridge, dumped last month's carton of milk into the trash, and got himself an ice-cold seltzer. Then he returned to his suitcases and, between gulps of bubbly, restored his collection of travel hardware to the concealed gun rack and deposited his laundry in the hamper. When he finished unpacking, Vic settled into an overstuffed chair by the picture window, drink and file folder in hand. For nearly ten minutes he sat, supremely content, enjoying the forest view and the comforting feeling of being safe. This room was the only place where he felt he could let down his guard—no looking out for the other guy, no putting on an act, no bullshit. Home.

Vic opened the file on his lap. Inside were dozens of stories he'd clipped from the New York papers during his stay in Florida. He had been on recuperative leave for the last few weeks, out of the action. But that didn't mean he couldn't plan his next job while recovering. Vic felt fit enough to rejoin the game and had already chosen his next opponent. He picked up one of the news articles and looked long and hard at the headline: "Latino Family Killer Strikes Again."

Vic liked the *New York Post*. Nothing subtle about their journalism. Good old-fashioned kick-'em-in-the-balls headlines: "Headless Body Found in Topless Bar." And they were thorough in their coverage of sensational crimes, the type of news Vic favored. It was indispensable to his work.

As he skimmed the clippings it occurred to him that, counting Dominic Torres and Cousin Isidro down in Florida, the Latino Family Killer would be his twenty-first hit. Jeffrey Dahmer would have been number fifteen if that had worked out. The manhunter currently known as Vic Tanner didn't like to think about that fiasco. The police had beaten him to Dahmer—his only failure. But fate had its own plan for Jeffrey, one involving a blunt instrument and a sordid prison lavatory. A truly fitting end for someone obsessed with ultimate control over other human beings.

The manhunter thought back on the twenty fallen monsters, the slain dragons. Each had been a unique experience to be savored like a fine wine.

There had been Greg Hewett, Mr. Clean. Two bullets through an open door. Hewett had been his baptism of fire and blood. He hoped Christine and Jennifer Vandemark rested easier after that execution.

The second hunt was for Jeff Falkner, a rapist-murderer out in California. Over a three-year period, Falkner had strangled eight women and left their bodies tied to lampposts along the highways of the Sunshine State and Oregon. The manhunter had tracked him down, talked his way into Falkner's house, and pumped two .38 slugs into the animal.

His third outing was up in Wyoming. People had been disappearing without a trace along Route 80. He had felt sure that someone was killing those people in the desolate 108-mile stretch between Salinas and Green River, leaving only their abandoned and stripped cars behind. He found out he was right when Ernest Hineman tried to make him victim number twenty-three. That had proved to be a costly mistake on Hineman's part. The relatively wet-behind-the-ears manhunter had put a bullet in Ernest's head and left him on the highway with a note pinned to his shirt, telling where Ernest's twenty-two victims were buried. The local police had taken this as a sort of personal affront. They set up a statewide dragnet for Hineman's killer that netted them zilch. Nothing worse than a sore loser.

Number four was a homicidal pederast in Chicago named Jay Parsons. The manhunter had strangled Parsons with his bare hands.

Then there was Norm Ballard, a second-rate Ed Gein who liked to waylay unwary travelers who happened by his out-of-the-way Nebraska farm. He'd sink their cars in a nearby bog and make household decorations from his victims' remains. It took nearly four months to hunt the maniac down. The killer stuck a knife in the manhunter's left shoulder, before Ballard's face was blown off with a .357 Magnum.

In Boston, the manhunter discovered a daisy chain of murders the police hadn't yet spotted as a series: eight stabbings on street corners over a four-year period. The wallet of each victim was missing, so robbery was the suspected motive. The hunter was going through microfilmed back issues of the Boston Globe when he stumbled upon the fact that one of these killings had occurred every six months. Searching for a common denominator, he uncovered the fact that all the victims had been alumni of Thomas Dewey High School, class of 1967. This clue eventually led him to Sylvester Gooden. When he cornered the killer, Gooden explained how the eight victims had bullied him unmercifully all through school. The manhunter slit Gooden's throat and left a note to the police clamped between Sylvester's teeth.

Seven and eight were the Helfer brothers, Dean and Todd. New Jersey state police knew these siblings had robbed and murdered nine small-business owners in the Newark area, but they couldn't prove it. The manhunter read the minds of the two men and acted as their judge, jury, and executioner. Regrettably, Todd Helfer managed to put a bullet into his executioner's leg a second before the avenger blew them both away with a shotgun. That was the first time the manhunter had required the services of the late lamented Dr. Lipston.

Karl Potter liked to lace children's aspirin with rat poison and sneak the bottles onto the shelves of San Francisco drugstores. The manhunter had managed to infiltrate the local FBI office and get a reading off one of the tampered-with bottles before all existing traces were obliterated by heavy-handed investigators in search of more tangible evidence. He had then tied Potter to a chair and force-fed him a bottle of his own medicine.

Abe Forrester, Dan Baker, and Jackson King considered themselves warlocks. They kidnapped children and sacrificed them to the devil after skinning them alive. It took the hunter two grueling months and several splendid leaps of logic to run them to ground in their Rocky Mountain retreat. The bodies of twenty-seven boys and girls, all under the age of ten, were later found on the site by the authorities. Forrester and King were also found, dead of gunshot wounds. Baker's body was eventually discovered about a mile from the retreat, slashed beyond recognition. The manhunter had escaped with no fewer than six knife wounds himself: Dan Baker had refused to die without a fight.

Wilma Dayton, a.k.a. Starr Windom, was the only woman the hunter had ever executed. He didn't regret it, but to this day the memory left a bad taste in his mouth.

Wilma had a nasty habit of picking up men in hotel bars, getting invited up to their rooms, and fixing them a drink laced with undiluted PCP. While the men bounced off the walls, Wilma helped herself to their billfolds. Three of her victims died of heart attacks, one jumped out his twenty-eighth-floor hotel-room window, another ran in front of a Mack truck screaming that snakes were after him. The manhunter crept up behind Wilma as she was preparing a special cocktail for him and put a dainty little hole in the back of her head with a .22 Beretta.

Lance O'Dell was a good-natured, helpful young man, fresh out of college. Everyone was sure he had a great future ahead of him and would go far. To this day, most of his old friends found it hard to believe that over a four-year period, Lance had raped and killed twenty-four women in five different states. Finding O'Dell had been a fluke, like Torres, not the result of hours and hours of homework. The manhunter had been relaxing in a bar when Lance came in, flushed from his latest kill, radiating pride in his accomplishments. The hunter had followed him out of the bar, stuck a gun in his ribs, and ordered Lance to take him to the site of his latest killing. At first Lance pretended not to understand what his kidnapper was talking about. But that changed when the hunter described in great detail O'Dell's most recent crime. They returned to where Lance had buried the victim, and the manhunter tortured his captive into writing a full confession and then beat him to death with a tree limb. The savagery of that execution bothered him sometimes. It must have been sparked by the duration of the close proximity to O'Dell.

Number fifteen was fourteen-year-old Daniel Seymour,

who liked to toss cinder blocks off overpasses through the windshields of cars on Los Angeles freeways. Ten people were killed by Danny's missiles. The police had tried to hush up the incidents, but the manhunter got wind of them by scanning the mind of an off-duty officer in a restaurant. He got the rest of what he needed from a hunk of cinder block investigators had failed to recover from one of the crime scenes. Then he visited Danny at his home while the boy's parents were out. Danny tried to jam a butcher knife into him, but the hunter wrenched it away and slit Danny's throat with it. He then explained his actions in a brief note, which ended with an apology for the mess he'd left behind.

Everything had been going pretty smoothly up until that point. Maybe it was because Danny Seymour had been such an easy kill. Maybe it was the boy's age. Or perhaps it was because the manhunter was getting tired. He'd been on the job for nearly five years by then. Something inside him made him decide to change the rules of the game. It had all become too easy. He decided to start handicapping himself.

When he tracked down Travis Stacy, an asylum escapee who was hiding deep in the Vermont woods, living off the land and what he could steal from the campers he murdered, the manhunter decided to give the guy an even break, even though the lunatic had butchered thirteen people in their sleep. The hunter didn't even pull his gun until after he informed Stacy that he was going to execute him. He waited until Travis had his shotgun in hand and was bringing it up to fire before rolling to the left and pumping two .45 bullets into the woodland maniac.

Jason Clarkson, a North Dakota mountain man, had

wiped out a family in New Hardec. He'd broken into their home and gunned them down one at a time, ending with the children. Clarkson felt the father had cheated him on a land deal. The state police had no luck tracking Clarkson through the Dakota Badlands into which he'd disappeared. The manhunter decided to give it a try, taking only a .38 pistol. It took him three weeks, on foot, to locate Clarkson. For two days after that, Jason Clarkson held his pursuer at bay, taking full advantage of the longer range of his hunting rifle. On the twenty-third night of the hunt, the avenger crept up behind the vigilant mountain man, whispered good-bye into his ear, and blew his brains out.

The manhunter sliced the odds against himself even finer when he went after Elmore Keefer, the Nevada cannibal who had come up with his own unique way to get around the high cost of beef. The hunter had only one bullet left in his gun when he confronted the shotgun-wielding Keefer. That was why he had to borrow Agent Levitt's gun before facing the two police officers standing between him and escape.

He'd had no weapon on him at all when he took on Torres and his trained gorilla.

Vic Tanner tossed back his last sip of seltzer. How could he possibly top the Torres killing? What would he have to do in New York to sweeten the victory this time? He wondered how close he could come to death without being claimed by that dark mistress.

17

JULY 15, 1996
WAR MEMORIAL PARK, WASHINGTON, D.C.

As Vida read through the file folder, Ira sat quietly on the park bench beside her. When she looked up, her eyes sparked with undisguised irritation at her low-key, cigar-smoking partner. "Why wasn't this file included in the records you sent home with me last night?"

Ira blew a number of smoke rings into the air, maddeningly taking his time, enjoying the moment. "Puts a whole different light on Vandemark, doesn't it? I held that info back because I was three years on the Vandemark case before I found out about it. Wanted you to grasp the bulk of the job before I laid this on you."

"You came across this information accidentally?"

"Yeah, I was getting nowhere tracking Vandemark. Thought getting a better idea about his past might give me a clearer understanding of the man, so I took a trip out to Strongville, Ohio, where David was born and where his parents were supposed to have died in an auto accident.

"Imagine my surprise when I found it was no car that killed Mr. and Mrs. Dwayne Vandemark. Town records stated that both husband and wife died of gunshot wounds. I went to police headquarters and got the whole story. Chief Romney remembered the case vividly. He was only a rookie when it happened.

"Apparently Dwayne Vandemark took to drinking when his business bellied up in 1966. He flipped out six months later and during a fight with his wife, pulled a gun and shot her in the heart. Then he ate the piece in front of his three-year-old son, David. Doctors claimed David had no memory of the killings. They thought it best to create the myth of the car crash. Back in 1966, they didn't know much about how the subconscious remembers things, even in cases of trauma-induced amnesia."

"Sure plays into Cruz's theory that Vandemark was somehow involved in his family's murders."

"Only if you're playing fast and loose with the facts."

"Have you had a psychological profile done on Vandemark?"

"Tried. The Bureau's shrinks do a pretty fancy song and dance, but they can't pigeonhole our boy the way they do your garden-variety psycho."

They sat in silence for a time, Vida seemingly lost in thought, mutely toying with a corner of the folder, Ira's eyes resting on the funereal expanse of the war memorial. Vida's voice, when at last she spoke, insinuated itself into the silence like wind rustling the branches of a tree. "That poor child."

Vida looked up to find Ira watching her, tension etched across his normally placid features. "Don't worry, Ira, I won't let my personal feelings get in the way. Sad story or not, I realize Vandemark's got to be stopped."

Ira nodded, relieved that Vida was so quick to put it together. He relaxed and turned once again toward the war memorial. After a few seconds he said, "My kid brother's name is on that wall."

Vida kept looking at him, unable to think of a single thing to say.

"If he had survived, he'd be about ten years older than Vandemark. In a lot of ways, they remind me of each other. That's what makes this case so hard for me sometimes."

"I didn't know. I'm sorry."

"Alan died more than twenty-five years ago. No reason to be sorry. I've cried all the tears for him I'm ever going to. I brought him up only because I want you to know why I'd like to take Vandemark alive. I've seen enough young men die in my time. And even though he's a monster, I believe this monster is living by his own personal code of honor. He's doing what he thinks is right."

"I suppose so."

"We'll bust him while he's still breathing, if he lets us. But you've got to realize that we may have to kill this man to bring him down. You're new at this and I've only got your word that you'll hold together when the time comes. You go soft on me, we may both end up dead."

Vida nodded her understanding. Ira blew a new set of smoke rings into the air.

"So what do we do with the rest of the day?" she asked.

Ira turned and beamed an impish smile at his companion. "We take the afternoon off, go home, and pack for a trip. Probably be gone at least a week. I've got us booked on a seven-ten flight tonight out of Baltimore International."

"That's kind of sudden, isn't it? What's happened?"

"Nothing yet. But I think I've figured out where Vandemark is going to surface next."

"Where's that?"

"Ever been to New York?"

PART TWO

Abattoir

He who spares the bad injures the good.

—*Publius Syrus*

18

Vic Tanner had forgotten how much he disliked New York City. No, make that *hated*. Getting stuck in bumper-to-bumper traffic as he inched his way across the George Washington Bridge was a blatant reminder. Too much dirt, way too much noise, and all that squirming and buzzing humanity. Vic, his hair and Vandyke dyed jet black, brown-tinted contacts in place, had packed the van last evening and was all set to leave first thing in the morning. But he decided that rushing off at the crack of dawn was a bad idea.

He was no longer Vic Tanner the actor. His wallet bulged with plastic and papers that showed the owner of this beat-up black van to be one Leroy De Carlo, a private eye from Chicago. His Illinois investigator's license was current, as was a temporary permit to work in New York State. He'd made sure every piece of ID had been appropriately aged, of course, as soon as it came off Vic Tanner's laser printer. Years of practice, together with the remarkable advances in desktop publishing, had given him all the capabilities needed to produce forgeries that would have fooled even the sharpest examiner. He was

proud of his craftsmanship. This Leroy De Carlo identity
would pass a computer check with flying colors. Vic marveled at the ease with which it was possible to access any
city or state's computer system and thus create a new citizen for them. Chicago had more than its share of private
investigators. Who would notice one more?

Leroy had his cover story ready. His research had
shown that the family murdered last week, the Menguellis, had no surviving relatives in the States. That made
them ideal for his needs. If anyone asked, Leroy De Carlo
was working for the late Hernando Menguelli's uncle
Manuel, who lived in a Chicago suburb. By the time they
could ascertain that no such uncle actually existed, Leroy
would have slipped comfortably into a new identity.

Yes, that part of the operation was completely in order.
And the Ford van was loaded with everything he would
need on this trip: a cache of weapons and clothes for
nearly every contingency, detailed maps of all five bor-
oughs, six spare sets of ID, a personal computer, wiretap-
ping equipment, case files, and dozens of other odds and
ends that might prove useful. The van was a three-
quarter-ton vehicle with a rebuilt 327-cubic-inch engine
bored out to 350, duel quads, and the best muffler money
could buy. Anyone seeing it on the streets would think it
was just another beat-up delivery truck—a perception
that would change radically if he chose to put the pedal
to the metal.

Leroy had neatly mapped out his strategy on this case.
This job looked as if it might be a breeze. All he'd have to
do is interview a few folks and get a good psychic reading
off one of the crime scenes, then make an educated guess
as to the next neighborhood the Latino Family Killer

would strike next, stake it out, and catch the sicko in the act. At least that was what Leroy was hoping. He already wanted to get out of New York in the worst way.

In truth, it wasn't the noise, air pollution, traffic jams, high prices, crime, hustle and bustle, or ambience of the Big Apple that bothered Leroy. It was the people. There were too God-awful many of them, all packed into too small a space. Like angry ants in a stirred-up anthill. Crowds are a telepath's worst enemy. Leroy hated them. Even when he consciously damped their input, he found the effort of dealing with large groups of people exhausting. Their maddeningly incessant mental chatter wore down his patience and goodwill. It was like having a small flying insect stuck in his ear. Practice had taught him how to endure the annoyance, but not with a smile.

Crowds were also a danger. When the input volume was lowered, so were Leroy's defenses. He had no way of knowing whether someone on a busy street was planning to stick a knife in him, slap on a pair of handcuffs, or pass him by unmolested. True, Leroy could focus on a single person in a group by deliberately zeroing in, but then everyone else was lost in the hubbub.

That was why many of his hunts had taken place in sparsely populated locales. Rule of thumb: Fewer people meant less grief. But he couldn't always pick his battles. There were other serial killers presently operating in more favorable locations, but none of them were taking out whole families at a time. Some temptations were worth the aggravation and risk. The trick was to get the job done and get out.

Traffic opened up some and Leroy jumped on the Harlem River Drive, heading toward the FDR. He got off at Thirty-fourth Street, found a vacant parking spot on Twenty-seventh off Park and squeezed into it. Having decided to go over the Quinoñes' file once more, he fished it out from under the seat.

The family of Angela Margarita Dolores Quinoñes had been the Slasher's first victims. Every other week in the seven weeks since then, with disturbing regularity, the killer had struck again, always during the second and fourth weeks of the month, but never on the same day. Always at night but never at the same hour and never twice in the same neighborhood. The two-week schedule and the ethnicity of his victims appeared to be this killer's only pattern.

Miss Quinoñes, who worked as an art director for a high-class fashion magazine, had lost two younger brothers and her parents to this mad butcher. She'd been spared only because she'd moved into her own apartment two years earlier. She was twenty-eight years old, had black hair and brown eyes, weighed 110 pounds, and stood five feet six. Leroy hadn't been able to locate a picture of Angela, so he was still entertaining the idea of a sexy Latin spitfire. He wasn't letting the fact that the lady's parents had immigrated from Cuba just before Fidel took over and that she had been born and raised in the United States get in the way of his little fantasy. Leroy skimmed through the rest of the data, then stashed the file back under the seat, hopped out of the van, and locked up.

Leroy had no worries about his wheels being there when he returned. He'd made sure that he wasn't in a tow-away zone and had armed his alarm system. Anyone who tried to check out what goodies the beat-up old van might contain would be greeted by an eardrum-splitting wail of protest. The siren would cut off after three minutes, and the system would rearm itself.

Even if the heist artist was blasé enough or stoned enough to ignore the alarm, he'd soon discover the ten-year-old van was practically impenetrable. Long hours had been put into reinforcing the doors and locks. Even a firefighter with the Jaws of Life would have had a tough time getting through all the reinforced paneling and bulletproof glass.

Angela lived in a fifth-floor walk-up on Twenty-seventh Street. But she wasn't in. Leroy didn't like this. It was nearly seven; she'd had plenty of time to get home from work. Was she out on a date? Could she possibly be out of town? A lot of Leroy's carefully planned scenario depended on locating this woman early in the game.

As luck would have it, the building's super was home, a short German man in his late fifties. He assured Leroy that Miss Quinoñes was not on vacation. He'd seen her only this morning, though he had no idea where she might be now. From the superintendent's mind Leroy learned that Angela sometimes had dinner at a neighborhood restaurant. The super hadn't volunteered this information because he didn't like this dark stranger's looks. This amused Leroy greatly. He wondered what the old coot would say when the dark stranger moved in with Angela Quinoñes.

On his way down the block Leroy caught sight of his reflection in a store window. He paused long enough to straighten his collar and brush his hair back with one hand. First impressions and all that.

Leroy spotted her near the back of the restaurant, eating alone. He knew instantly it was Angela, although she was too far away to get a reading. The image of the Latin spitfire vanished, replaced instantly by the real flesh-and-blood Angela Quinoñes.

Angela was stylishly dressed, which was no surprise, considering her line of work. Regular workouts were apparently a part of her routine. Taut, graceful muscles played along her arms as she cut something on her plate. Her hair was short and puckishly playful, but that was the only playful thing about her. The haircut accentuated her dark, thickly lashed eyes, serious oval face, and long, elegant neck. Her lips were full and sensuous, but it was her eyes Leroy was drawn to.

Every time those eyes looked up, Leroy was struck by the overwhelming sadness in them. It was a quiet undercurrent, something she was trying to keep hidden beneath a cool facade. But Leroy had trained himself to see things that most people missed. He saw the sorrow and then had a hard time seeing anything else.

After a few moments spent observing his subject, Leroy decided to make his entrance. Step softly with this one, he warned himself. Angela Quinoñes was like cracked crystal: beautiful to look at, but likely to shatter if not handled gently.

Leroy made his way to the back of the restaurant like a man who knew exactly where he was going. Angela treated him to an icy inspection when he arrived at her table.

Realizing she thought this was a clumsy pickup attempt, Leroy promptly launched into his spiel. "Good evening. My name's Leroy De Carlo, Miss Quinoñes. I'm a private investigator from Chicago." He showed her his license. "I was hoping I could talk to you. I'm in . . . the . . ."

Leroy let his voice trail off. He didn't understand what was happening. All he could do was stand there, staring at Angela Quinoñes, a comically exaggerated look of surprise on his face. He was making a Herculean effort to connect with her, but nothing was coming to him. It was embarrassing. This had never happened to him before, and he wasn't quite sure what to do. How was this possible? What was there about Angela Quinoñes that kept him from being able to see into her mind?

19

"Are you all right?" inquired Angela, her glacial stare softening into an expression of concern.

The man who had interrupted her dinner rubbed his forehead and smiled ruefully. "Yes. Been on the road all day. Guess I'm feeling a little light-headed. Mind if I sit down? I really do need to speak to you."

"About what?"

"I'm investigating the Latino Family Murders."

Some part of her had known what he was going to say. It had been two months since her family was killed, but his words touched a wound that was open and raw. Angela could feel anger and pain well up immediately. More questions! How many times had she answered the same questions? Her father, mother, and brothers were still dead, still unable to rest easy. The questions would never bring them back, and they weren't going to help catch the killer.

So why put up with this nonsense? Hit the road, Mr. Question Man. I don't want to play this game anymore. Leave me alone, so I can mourn my dead and maybe somehow find my way back to a life that doesn't include a daily crying jag. Give me a chance to heal. Go away!

But Angela looked up at the man with her sad eyes, as he stood waiting respectfully, and said, "Have a seat."

Angela had to ask his name again. De Carlo. Leroy De Carlo. The name sounded Spanish, but the accent was strictly midwestern. He quickly explained that he'd been hired by the well-to-do uncle of one of the Slasher's latest victims. Dissatisfied with the results of the NYPD investigation, he had hired De Carlo to help find the murderer. Leroy said he'd had some success with a couple of similar cases in the Midwest. That was why he had been called in.

Signaling a waiter, Leroy ordered a beer for himself and another glass of white wine for her. When he turned his attention back to Angela he seemed unsure what to say next. Angela couldn't put her finger on it exactly, but she felt that this interview wasn't going at all the way Leroy had planned it. But why? She was cooperating with him, wasn't she?

Finally he said, "It's like this, Angela. I'm here in a strange city, on a case that's two months cold. I've got no useful leads, so I need all the help I can get. I'm good at what I do, but I'm no Superman."

"What can I add that you don't already know from police reports and newspaper articles? I assume you've already gone over that material?"

"Over and over. And you know what? I didn't find anything that would clue me in on who this Slasher is. So I've got to take another approach completely. When I can't get a lead on a killer, I try to find out more about the victims. That's why I came to see you."

Angela digested that for a few moments. "I can understand how that would work in a conventional murder case. But this Slasher seems to pick his victims at random. He's a madman, a monster. He can't possibly have had a sane reason for killing my family or any of the others. None of the victim families knew each other. There wasn't any connection between them."

"Correction: there wasn't any connection between them that anyone's managed to uncover. Even a lunatic works within a framework of some sort. If this killer were as random and scattershot as the papers like us to think, he would have screwed up by now and been caught."

"I don't understand how you can say that. Didn't David Berkowitz, the Son of Sam, operate like that? Look how long it took the police to catch him."

"Berkowitz was different. He was running around the streets, shooting people in parked cars. It was the spur-of-the-moment nature of his crimes that made him so hard to track. But you see, the Slasher is quite another matter. He knows who his victims are. It's no accident, for instance, that all of his victims are Hispanic. They've been chosen because of their ethnicity. He also takes them out in their homes. That's important. In order to do that, he's got to have checked out the situation carefully before going in. No one, not even a madman, breaks into a strange building to kill without first knowing the layout. My guess is that he'd been inside their homes at least once before he murdered those poor people."

This caught Angela up short. "But . . . the police never said anything like that."

"Not because they haven't thought of it. But they've got to be closemouthed about what they say. I don't have that problem, since there're no newspaper reporters hanging on my every word."

"I see. Then what you'd like from me is anything I can remember about my family that might tie them in with the other victims."

"Exactly. It'd be a great help if you could tell me all about your father, mother, and brothers—give me a family history. Later on I'll contact the relatives of each of the other victim families, and maybe some connection will surface that the police have missed. I have more time to spend on this one case than they do. And I've got a fresh outlook. I haven't been living with this tragedy for two months already. That's my edge. It's worked for me before."

Angela wondered whether she was up to the task of talking about her family to the extent Leroy De Carlo was describing. Could she handle it? It was going to be hard; of that she was certain. She knew she couldn't do it here, in the restaurant."

"Let's go to my apartment."

⋙⋘

Angela watched De Carlo survey her abode. His scrutiny made her feel self-conscious about the trendy high-tech furniture. Until now it had never seemed quite so out of place to her. Old New York surrounding Space Age chairs and end tables. She'd thought the look was eclectic but suddenly it seemed merely pretentious.

This one was definitely an investigator. He didn't look at things, he examined them. On the other hand, he didn't exactly fit her expectations of a private eye. Someone cynical and a bit unsavory. A low-level hood with a license that enabled him to work at unorthodox law enforcement. Leroy wasn't like that at all. In fact, he seemed almost shy and studious. "Bookish" was maybe a better word. Reticent. She had the distinct impression that he wasn't comfortable in her presence. He'd hesitated visibly at the suggestion of coming up to her place, a fact she found amusing. Experience had taught her that most men would leap at the chance to get her up here alone.

But Angela didn't have any mistaken impression that this Leroy was some sort of a pushover intellectual with a weak handshake. She watched the way he moved, and she had stolen a couple of quick glances at his eyes while he dealt with the waiter. There was steel inside this man. He hid it well, but it was there.

She offered him a drink and was surprised when he asked for soda. Angela got herself another glass of white wine, and they settled down in the living room.

"Where should I start?"

Leroy said, "Tell me about the different places your family lived while you were growing up. Talk about your childhood. Let the memories flow."

Angela was surprised at how easy it was for her to do this. She began by telling Leroy about growing up in the South Bronx. Her dad had worked as a janitor in a pharmaceutical lab. It hadn't been easy for him the first ten or so years in this country. His English was poor and his Cuban college degree didn't mean anything here. He eventually got a job at Elmhurst Hospital in Queens and moved his family to Flushing. Her parents had remained in that second-floor apartment until their death. The place had always been home to Angela: welcoming, warm, comforting. She found it hard to believe their lives had ended in such horror. Angela had not been able to return to the apartment after the murders. Friends had disposed of the family's possessions. She'd saved only a handful of mementos: her father's camel-hair brushes, some of her mother's jewelry, a few photos.

As she talked, Angela noticed that Leroy was a good listener, leaning forward in his seat, nodding, occasionally asking a question, but willing to let her go her own way undirected. She began to realize this talk was exactly what she needed. Her grief had been bottled up for too long. It was beginning to fester. And now Leroy had given her this great gift: an opportunity to cleanse herself, heart and soul. This was her chance to remember, to speak of the warmth and kindness of her family. Tears came, but they didn't interrupt her recital. Angela merely blew her nose, wiped her eyes, and continued. These tearful moments didn't seem to disturb De Carlo in the least, so he didn't interrupt Angela's therapeutic purging. Yes, he was a good listener, all right. About the best she'd ever met.

Angela spoke of family weekend jaunts to Jones Beach. Of trips to the Brooklyn Botanical Gardens. How she had loved that beautiful oasis in the middle of her concrete and asphalt world. She spoke warmly of a vacation in Atlantic City before it became the East Coast's great gambling mecca. She and her brother had bicycled along the boardwalk and sampled the amusements. It had been fun, but there had also been drama—a shark alert that kept everyone out of the water. Angela remembered sitting on the beach with her family, carefully scanning the ocean for some sign of a fin, but never spotting one. Those two weeks had been one of the high points of her childhood, a taste of what growing up could be like outside the big city. It was the only vacation her family had ever been able to afford.

That thought changed the course of Angela's reminiscing. Yes, there had been lots of fun, but there were also hard times. Most of her young life had been spent in a lower-middle-class neighborhood. There hadn't been a lot of luxuries, but the basic necessities of life were usually there.

Angela was six when her parents decided they could afford more children. They may have been the only couple in America to successfully use the rhythm method. By the time she'd reached her eighth birthday she had two baby brothers. Then three days before her ninth birthday, her father was laid off at the hospital. There had been cutbacks. Those with the least seniority were let go, with a promise of being called back if things got better. Unemployment insurance ran out after six months; there were no jobs to be had. Sometimes the family skipped meals. Old clothes that should have been tossed out were repaired or altered. Angela remembered the sadness in her father's voice when he announced that they would have to go on welfare. It was almost more than his pride could bear.

This bleak existence continued for three months until the miracle happened: Elmhurst Hospital had called. Her father got his job back, and life righted itself and continued on an even keel for many years.

Angela's college board scores were good enough to win her a Regents scholarship. She had used it to realize her dreams of an art-school education, a bachelor's degree from the School of Visual Arts. After that came a series of jobs at small newspapers, magazines, and ad agencies, doing comps, speccing type, and calligraphy.

Then, three years ago, Angela landed a part-time job at the fashion magazine she now worked at. That was her big break. A year later she was a full-time art director with the financial freedom to get her own place. A haven all her own. That was why she wasn't living at home when tragedy struck. Again the tears came. But this time Angela could not continue. She buried her face in her hands and sobbed uncontrollably. Angela wasn't aware of Leroy getting out of his chair, coming over, and sitting beside her until he gently touched her shoulder. The next thing Angela knew, she had her face pressed against his chest, her entire frame racked with shuddering sobs. As she fought to regain her composure, she continued weeping, but her convulsive sobs began to subside until they sounded more like hiccups. All this time Leroy held her lightly and patiently patted her on the back, whispering that it was okay; let it all come out.

When she had settled down, Leroy resumed his seat without fanfare or explanation. He asked next about Angela's mother.

Angela spoke with deep feeling of Rosanna Quinoñes, describing how their relationship had always been special, much more so than that of many mothers and daughters she knew. Not even Angela's rebellious teenage years had been able to strain the special love they felt for each other. Rosanna was a friend and a confidante. Angela noted how Leroy's interest seemed to quicken when she related how, at age ten, she had taken a terrible fall off her bike and struck her head. She had lain unconscious for nearly two days in a hospital bed. Rosanna Quiñoñes had never left her side during that time. Angela thought it a bit peculiar that De Carlo seemed more interested in her injury than in the story itself. She couldn't understand what bearing her concussion had on Leroy's investigation. But Angela shrugged it off, deciding private eyes made all sorts of strange connections that others didn't see. She was deep in remembering her mother and wouldn't let a little quirky curiosity distract her.

Rosanna Quiñoñes had remained at home until Tomás and Jorge, Angela's brothers, had entered high school. Then she had found work in a secretarial pool. It was the first paying job she'd ever had. Angela was so proud and pleased for her. The extra income brought a few amenities into the house, such as color television and a new fridge. At that time it had looked as if life was destined to get better and better. No one in the family had any major problems. The boys were doing well in school. Her dad had worked his way up the hospital's custodial ladder and was now a custodial manager. Mother loved her work. Angela had a boyfriend and her job at the magazine. The boyfriend didn't work out, but the job did. Life wasn't perfect, but it was mighty close. Close enough to suit Angela.

Then the Latino Family Killer struck, and with blinding speed everything—*everything*—was gone. Wiped out in the blink of an eye.

This time Angela didn't break down in tears at this mention of the murders. She realized that the long healing process had begun. There was pain in Angela's eyes. And sorrow. But there was also something new that until this moment she hadn't allowed herself to feel. A something much healthier than the futility she had been suffering. That something was anger.

Angela realized then how much she wanted the murderer caught and punished for the cruelty he'd inflicted, the lives he'd shattered. The dreams he had snuffed out.

At that moment she decided she would help Leroy De Carlo in any way she could.

Up until that point Angela had been speaking quietly, as if to herself, almost completely lost in her own thoughts. She glanced over at Leroy to find that he was perusing the assortment of framed photographs on the end table next to his chair. He had one in his hand. Though she couldn't see the picture itself, Angela recognized it by its frame.

"This your boyfriend?" Leroy asked.

"Was."

"Was?"

"We broke up. He's been in prison for over a year, but that's a different sad story."

"What happened?" Leroy asked as he returned the picture to its place on the table.

"His name is Jeffrey Parker. He was a stockbroker, a real player on Wall Street. Jeff was . . . flamboyant, exciting to be with. Such gambling can be very seductive, Mr. De Carlo. We were going to be married this year. But things went bad and we ended it. A couple of months later he was arrested in the men's room at his office. Cocaine. Third time busted. Such a terrible waste. I've cried myself out for Jeffrey, though."

Leroy got to his feet and wandered over to a window. With his back to her he said, "Life has been pretty rough for you."

Angela didn't answer.

De Carlo glanced at his wristwatch and announced, "Look, I'd better get going. Thank you for all the help you've given me. What you've told me might come in quite handy."

"I'd like to help in any other way that I can, Mr. De Carlo," she said. "If there's anything else I can do, please give me a call. I want to hear how you're doing with your investigation. Where can I get in touch with you?"

"Haven't gotten settled yet. I'll see if I can find a place near one of the airports. I understand rents are cheaper out that way."

Angela looked at the clock on the wall and was shocked to find it was nearly two-thirty. Had she been talking all that time? It would be sheer hell getting up in the morning. But that wasn't important right now.

"Listen," she said, "you're going to have a terrible hassle finding a hotel at this hour. Why don't you use my couch? Find a place tomorrow."

Leroy smiled wanly, accepted the offer, and thanked her, then turned back toward the window.

Angela wondered what he was thinking. Inviting strange men to spend the night wasn't her usual style. But this Leroy De Carlo was different.

It was obvious he hadn't taken her invitation to mean anything more than what it was: an offer to use the sofa. She was pleased to find her assessment of De Carlo verified. She was also relieved that he was staying. After all the talk of her family, this apartment would have seemed very large and empty tonight without someone else around.

Angela disappeared momentarily and returned with

sheets, a blanket, and a pillow. She informed Leroy that the couch folded out. He took the bedding and thanked her. Then Angela made what sounded to her like a couple of awkward comments about the lateness of the hour and the early-morning agony of hearing an alarm clock go off. Leroy nodded understandingly and they said good night.

⌇⌇⌇⌇⌇

Alone in her room, Angela found that sleep wasn't going to come easily despite the late hour. She lay in bed, listening to the sounds of Leroy making up the sofa in the other room. She sensed, with an unshakable certainty, that she could trust this Leroy De Carlo. She knew she wouldn't have someone trying to sneak into her bed tonight. This one wouldn't do anything to hurt her. Sometimes it happened that way—a few hours with a person and she felt that she'd known him forever.

All this talk of the dead had reminded Angela how fragile life was. Her own mortality weighed heavily on her. It was a comfort having this guardian angel for one night, standing watch at her door, ready to drive off any demons that might materialize out of the darkness.

⌇⌇⌇⌇⌇

After making up the couch, Leroy returned to the living-room window, which overlooked the constantly bustling city. He needed to take a walk, but decided against it. The tension, he decided, would subside on its own. He'd drift off to sleep eventually.

Usually when he started a job, the first thing he did was find a home base. Leroy's preferred method of operation involved making the acquaintance of a female relative of one of his prey's victims. This gave him access to a cornucopia of information that never got into the papers, as well as a reason for hanging around.

With his gift it wasn't hard for him to insinuate himself into someone's life. When you knew exactly what someone wanted to hear, it was a snap to say the right things in just the right tone of voice. He'd taken some acting lessons along the way to prepare for his Vic Tanner identity. They'd been invaluable.

He tried to play fair with the temporary liaisons he formed. Leroy never promised them anything and avoided sleeping with them unless it was absolutely unavoidable, or irresistible. This never sat quite right with him afterward, but he rationalized that the ends justified the means. After all, he was going to avenge their loss and tie up those loose ends so they'd be able to get on with their lives, still believing that there was some justice in this world.

When time came for him to leave it wasn't hard for him to arrange things so that it was his hostess's idea. As a result he departed on the best of terms, leaving behind fond memories of something that was sweet but that would never have worked out.

But this Angela. That lady was the source of his current agitation. She was like no one he had ever met. Leroy concluded that his inability to read her mind was merely some type of physiological abnormality, most likely a result of the head injury she had suffered as a child. Angela Quiñoñes probably wasn't the only person whose mind he couldn't look into. She was merely the first he'd ever met face to face. There was nothing supernatural or scary about it. It was unusual, but there was a simple explanation for it.

Angela herself was another matter. How had she managed to lose everyone near and dear to her and keep from going to pieces? She hadn't crawled into a bottle or taken to anesthetizing the pain with pills or street drugs.

Over the years Leroy had met a lot of people who were either coping or not coping with loss. He had seen plenty of folks lose themselves in self-pity and let their lives go down the drain. He'd also watched people go to the other extreme—total denial: I'm okay. I can handle it. What pain?

When these people went to pieces, they did so in spectacular fashion. You could only hold it in so long before you explode, but some fools refused to believe that. They were nearly as pitiful as the ones who drank away their future.

Angela Quinoñes was something else again. A fighter. The lady was facing her grief head on. He marveled at the way she had talked about her family tonight. Leroy had gone through this routine with other bereaved relatives, scanning their thoughts as they gave him verbal nuggets to work with. But Angela had given it all, without his having to pry. She had exposed her entire life for him to see, in the hope that it would help catch her family's killer. It couldn't have been easy for her. Those tears had been real. But they had eventually stopped, to be replaced by a look of immutable determination. Angela wanted the Slasher stopped. And she had the will and strength to help him do it.

Yes, she was quite a woman. Strength, beauty, brains, even talent. Leroy's eyes widened: he was surprised at the direction of his thoughts. Would you listen to yourself, pal? You're talking yourself into a Madonna obsession. So cool it. Remember, you'll only be in town long enough to get the job done. Don't turn the fact that you can't see into her mind into any big deal. Sure it's been nice talking to someone in a normal, everyday fashion, no mind-reading involved. Just don't let the experience turn you all soft and romantic.

Leroy De Carlo, or whatever your name is, you've got a mission in life. I know that sounds corny, but that's the way it is. No room in your life for a lady. Not even her. So nip any silly ideas you might have in the bud, fella. Understand? Understood. Get it? Got it. Good.

He removed his contact lenses, climbed in between the fresh sheets, and turned off the light. When he looked up at the ceiling, he saw its expanse was illuminated by a streetlight, but he could feel himself begin to drift off almost as soon as his head hit the pillow. That's how it was with him and sleep. Nothing, nothing, and then he was sandbagged by total oblivion. The last conscious thought he remembered was that if there'd been room for a woman in this chaos he called his life, Angela Margarita Dolores Quiñoñes could very easily have been the . . .

20

Angela woke before her alarm went off. She pulled on a robe and went to check on her house guest. She was amazed to discover him propped up on his elbows, looking back at her. Leroy nodded good morning. Angela did the same and vanished into the bathroom.

As she showered, Angela wondered how she might help De Carlo with his investigation. She gingerly tested her newfound determination. It held firm. A night's rest hadn't shaken her resolve to become involved. Before drifting off to sleep she'd worried that morning would find her fretting about the stand she'd committed herself to the previous night. But that wasn't the case at all. Angela was honestly looking forward to . . . to what? The adventure? She'd wrapped herself up for too long in a cocoon of solitude. The time had come to plunge back into the world of the living. No more hiding, she told herself. Let something besides your own pain **touch** you again.

The first thing that touched Angela was a grim dose of reality. Leroy was up and about in the kitchen, humming while helping himself to a cup of coffee, courtesy of her Space Age Make-Your-Coffee-Before-You're-Awake machine. He wasn't wearing the sport coat he'd had on last evening, so Angela had a good long look at the shoulder holster he was wearing. It contained a large, nasty-looking flat black pistol.

Angela had never had anything to do with guns. The thought of them made her nervous. She'd seen policemen on the street carrying guns, and plenty of people on television, of course. But her personal experience with firearms began and ended there. Rather remarkable, when you consider that her family had lived in New York. And not in the ritziest sections. Yet her father never had one and she'd never run with any crowd tough enough to carry pieces. Angela was momentarily embarrassed by this innocence. It made her feel strangely defensive about how sheltered her life had been. Leroy was completely relaxed despite the firearm he carried. It was there, a part of him. He wasn't toting it to prove anything to anyone. He seemed hardly aware of it. A tool of the trade. Nothing more.

Angela decided to be cool and ignore it. After all, she was a streetwise New Yorker, not easily shocked. Besides, she didn't want Leroy to think she'd scare this easily. Act blasé, that was the answer to this particular etiquette dilemma.

"Good morning," she said as she entered the kitchen.

Don't look at the gun. It won't bite you if you don't look at it.

Leroy glanced up from his cup and replied, "Mornin'. Want some java?"

"Yes. Thanks."

"Got any sugar around here?"

"In the cupboard above the sink."

Omigod! I almost said "In the gun above the sink"! You're looking! Stop! Look somewhere else! Say something quick!

"I've been thinking about how I might be of some help to you," she said.

"So have I. How's your Spanish?"

"Fluent. How's yours?"

"Pathetic. From the reports I've gone through, it looks like my best bet for a second interview is a Mrs. Vallejo. Her brother and his family were the Slasher's second set of victims. Newspaper reports said she doesn't speak English."

"Then I'll act as your interpreter. I get off work at six. You can meet me at the office or a restaurant. Then maybe we can go shoot her after some dinner. Do you like Italian? There's a place just . . . just . . ."

Shoot her after some dinner?

That did it. Her composure was in tatters.

Don't look at the gun! Maybe he didn't notice. If you ignore it, maybe it will go away. Don't look! You're looking! He's going to see!

Leroy smiled broadly, got up from the table, and walked out to the living room. He returned a moment later with his sport coat on and buttoned up.

"Yes, Italian would be fine. What'd you say the name of this eatery was?"

"La Bella Pasta."

"Sounds a bit uptown to me."

"It is. But the food's good."

Noticing the clock, Angela jumped up with coffee in hand and took off at a dead run in the direction of her bedroom. "Omigosh! I gotta dash! Going to be late."

❧❧❧

The smile lingered on Leroy's face as he watched Angela roar out of the kitchen. A little tension in the air this morning. That was okay. Kind of nice, in fact.

It was also a reminder that Angela Quinoñes wasn't a player. Keep that in mind, De Carlo. Use her on the interviews. She might even be handy for some other assorted bits of business. But remember, she's a noncombatant. Keep the lady out of the front lines.

❧❧❧

Leroy had finished his coffee and was getting ready to take off when Angela reemerged from the bedroom dressed and nearly ready to face the day. De Carlo had to admit she looked great. Keep your mind on business, Leroy.

"I'll be going," he said.

"Don't you want some breakfast?" asked Angela.

"Thanks, but no. I'll grab something on the way. I have quite a few things to do before I meet you tonight."

"Okay. Well, uh, you be careful out there. Didn't they used to say that on one of the cop shows?"

"*Hill Street Blues*, I think. See you later."

"Yeah, bye."

Leroy was on his way down the stairs when Angela called out to him. As he turned, glancing up the stairwell, she simply said, "Catch!"

The set of keys arced neatly through the air into Leroy's hands. He stared at them in confusion for a moment, then at Angela. She seemed more than a bit agitated and said hurriedly, "The round key's to the front door. The other two are for this one up here. There's no reason for you to hang around the street waiting for me to get off work. I'll meet you here."

She did a fast about-face, disappeared into the apartment, closed the door behind her, and sagged against it. Why had she done that? Why had she given this stranger the keys to the kingdom? Her kingdom . . .

And she could have sworn Leroy's eyes had been brown last night.

⋘⋗⋙

On the landing, Leroy was still gawking at the keys in his hand. Of course he was well aware of what was happening. Leroy had used his telepathic powers to finesse his way into a number of young ladies' hearts and habitats.

Trouble was, this time Leroy wasn't playing any mind games. He hadn't finessed anything with Angela Quinoñes. He couldn't: her mind was as unfathomable as the ocean to him. Try as he might, he wasn't able to pick up a single thought. And Leroy wasn't even trying to charm her. He was simply being himself. He'd written off the possibility of staying at her apartment. So why had she tossed him the keys? This question, and the accompanying realization that he wasn't exactly in control here, made Leroy uneasy.

Stuffing the keys in his pocket, he continued down the stairs. It didn't feel right this time around. Staying with Angela Quinoñes would prove to be a mistake. By the time he reached the street, Leroy knew he wasn't going to be able to pin down immediately what was bothering him about the arrangement, so he decided to forget it, at least for the moment. He could always worry about it when he had some free time. For now, he would go with the flow, keep his mind clear. He had work to do, and if he didn't keep his head clear on this job he was likely to get it lopped off.

Moving to an East Side parking lot spared Leroy's van from the towing hook. Once he'd gotten settled, Leroy climbed in back, shaved with an electric razor, and rapidly changed clothes and identities, donning a gray three-piece suit of the sort that a Justice Department lawyer would wear. Smiling, Leroy decided that Jason Colson could go with blue eyes.

Shit! The smile faded as Leroy remembered and reached for the contact lens case in his breast pocket. Had Angela noticed? Probably. He'd have to stick with blue eyes from here on. It didn't matter anyway. Even with the shiny black hair, he didn't think anyone would buy his Hispanic act under close scrutiny. Besides, those contacts were damned uncomfortable.

Jason picked up the *New York Times* and the *Post* and had a leisurely breakfast at a nearby coffee shop. Nothing new in the papers about the Slasher, so Jason decided to enjoy his meal without any further thought of the case. Sitting there, he absentmindedly flexed his leg, the one that still carried Ira Levitt's bullet. It felt a little stiff, but thoroughly trustworthy. For a week after returning to Willow Jason had started each morning with a long walk up into the forested hills behind his home. Each day the trek had become easier and longer. At midweek he had started jogging each afternoon. Now the limb felt up to anything he might have to challenge it with. A good thing, too. The Slasher was probably set to strike again next week. Only Jason was hoping to put that joker out of business before then.

❧❧❧❧

New York City was going all out to crack the Latino Family Murders. Nothing was too good for the task force in charge of the case. That was why they were headquartered at One Police Plaza. No squalid little precinct station house for them. It was first-class treatment all the way. After all, the investigation of a case of this notoriety was as much a media event as the crime.

Jason Colson got directions in the lobby of the monolithic steel, brick, and glass structure, rode up in the elevator, and was greeted by a grizzled old desk sergeant at the door of the task force's office. The officer sat behind a battered gray metal desk decorated only with a phone and a nameplate proclaiming him to be Sergeant Turpin. The man looked Colson up and down, sizing him up. "What can I do for you?" he asked.

Handing the sergeant his credentials, Jason announced with crisp efficiency, "Jason Colson, Justice Department. I'm here about the Latino Family Murders, Sergeant."

"Yeah, someone from your office called yesterday, saying we should expect you."

Jason didn't bother to correct the man: Jason himself had called from Willow. It was a lot easier to pierce the security veil if one called ahead. The unexpected visitor was always an object of suspicion.

Sergeant Turpin handed Jason back his papers and

asked, "What interest does the Justice Department have in these killings? This is a local murder case. Nothing federal about it."

"All of the Slasher's victims have been Hispanic. It's possible this killer has violated his victims' civil rights."

"Ya gotta be kiddin'!"

"I know how it sounds, but this case is getting national media attention, and the attorney general's office wants to have a backup plan in place in the event the local case doesn't hold up in court."

"Hell, you ain't got to worry about the city's case not floatin'. You're wasting your time here, not to mention the taxpayers' money."

"Listen, Sergeant, I know this civil rights investigation is just gilding the lily. I think even my superiors know it. But they want to cover their butts, so give me a break, eh? I'm a working stiff like you, just doing what I'm told. Okay?"

The officer thought it over and finally decided this Colson character was all right. Maybe he *was* a lawyer, but Turpin didn't have to hold that against him. The sergeant excused himself, got on the horn, spoke briefly to someone, and then told Jason to go see Lieutenant Nyberg in room 1107.

As Jason walked down the hall, he exhaled a sigh of relief. The old skills were working smoothly. His gift had shown him exactly what to say to Turpin. Meeting Angela had thrown his confidence a bit. But dealing with Turpin had reassured him that Ms. Quiñones was definitely the exception rather than the rule.

Lieutenant Philip Nyberg was a thin man in his midforties, with pinched features and wavy blond hair. As

Jason entered the room, Nyberg looked up from the papers on his desk and muttered, "More Feds. That's just what I need. As if this case weren't enough of a ball buster."

"Other federal agents? Who are they?" asked Jason.

"Two FBI agents. They're here investigating some kind of related matter that they're being really tight-assed about."

They were just "Feds" to Nyberg; Jason couldn't pick up their names. "I promise to stay out of your hair as best I can. I just want to review your case file to see if the federal government should pursue a civil rights violation case against your Slasher."

"Civil rights violation?"

"Yeah. You remember how they nailed the Ku Klux Klansmen who murdered those freedom marchers back in the sixties?"

Nyberg scratched at his jaw. "Sure. They charged them with that after the murder charges were dismissed. But there's no chance of that happening here. You should see the physical evidence we've got."

"Well, if you let me go over your files, I'll report that to my boss and I'm out of here. Okay?"

"Fine by me. Far be it from me to stand in the way of justice."

Jason knew he was taking a chance entering the beast's lair like this. He could feel it gently stirring in its sleep. No matter. The gamble had paid off and he felt invigorated by the danger. And the Justice Department cover had been sheer genius, if he had to say so himself. There was a good chance the FBI was already in on the case, so posing as one of their agents was out of the question. But to come in as a Justice Department lawyer, probing a possible civil rights violation, was perfect. It threw people off-balance with its air of screwy bureaucratic illogic.

Nyberg got up from his desk, walked to the door, and pointed down the hall. "Last door on your left. That's where you'll find the Slasher file. Knock yourself out. Oh, by the way, one of the Feds is going over it now. Don't trip over each other."

Jason thanked Lieutenant Nyberg, promised once again to be gone as soon as possible, and strolled down the hall. The last room on the left. The door was closed. Jason politely knocked before walking in.

He had been half expecting to be greeted by some throwback to J. Edgar Hoover's glory days: crew cut, humorless, dressed in a dark blue suit. Jason was used to dealing with lantern-jawed local police, some lowlifes, a few bereaved relatives, and then eventually his prey. Serial murderers seldom turned out to be beautiful people. But this case, so far, had certainly been a surprise. And a very pleasant one at that. Too bad everyone involved with this affair couldn't be this lovely.

A young woman looked up from the file, a quizzical expression on her pretty face.

Jason smiled and said, "You must be one of the Feds Nyberg was telling me about. I'm Jason Colson, Justice Department."

"Vida Johnson, FBI. Nyberg certainly doesn't think much of us, does he?"

"Locals always hate Federals. It's tradition. How you doing?"

"Grimly slogging through it. There's some really brutal stuff in here. Too bad there's no death penalty in New

York right now. If anyone deserves to fry, it's this baby. What's Justice's interest in the case?"

Jason smoothly recited his cover story and reiterated his bogus views on his mission. A quick scan of Vida's head showed she was buying all of it. She handed him a hefty section of the thick file that she'd already finished with and said, "You might as well start with the crime scene material and forensic reports. A mountain of paperwork has been created on this case. This file isn't even a tenth of it. The police compiled this abridged version to save me some time and keep me out of their way."

"Thoughtful of them. Nyberg said there were two of you on this case. Where's your partner?"

"Ira? He's off doing some legwork."

Ira? Ira Levitt!

Vida, preoccupied, didn't see her companion start as her partner's full name echoed through the corridors of his mind.

What the hell is Levitt doing here? Colson wondered. Then he realized that the answer to that question was obvious: He's after my ass. The same way I'm after the Slasher's. But how did he know I'd be here?

Jason ran through some logical possibilities and then remembered thinking that there were other serial killers operating in more favorable locations than New York, but none of them were taking out whole families at a time. Some temptations were worth the aggravation and risk.

Ira Levitt was getting to know his prey a little too well, as far as Jason Colson was concerned. The FBI agent had anticipated David Vandemark's next target and beaten him to it. But how much did Levitt know? Was it relatively safe for Colson to continue this hunt? Vida Johnson would know, and Jason could find out if he asked the right questions. It didn't matter that Vida probably wouldn't talk, even to a fellow Fed.

Jason leaned across the table and said, "Nyberg tells me you're working on a pretty hush-hush case. Anything interesting?"

Vida put down the paper she was reading, looked him right in the eye, and replied, "Very. But I can't talk about it. Orders, you know." She then attempted to turn her attention back to the file, but her thoughts were elsewhere, just as Jason had hoped. He read her thoughts clearly: Boy, would Colson be surprised how interesting this case really is. Tracking down Vandemark is . . .

All the facts came dancing out of Vida's mind, whirling in circles, faster and faster like dancers in a wild tarantella, until Jason felt exhausted examining them.

Pretending to inspect his section of the file, Jason listened intently as Vida mentally reviewed the case. After a while she tired of playing "What if Colson knew this?" and returned to the job at hand. But she had spilled enough to let Jason know where he stood. Now his only worry was that Levitt might walk in and recognize him before he'd read through the file.

He decided to take the direct approach. "When is your partner coming back? I'd like to get his view on this case too."

Without looking up from her work, Vida said, "He's not. We're going to meet uptown for lunch."

Another quick read told Jason she was telling the truth. It also showed that Vida was beginning to take a dislike to this nosy lawyer. Okay, he could live with that, for now. The future would take care of itself; he was more

concerned with the present—especially in regard to Ira
Levitt. Vida was not expecting her partner to return to
One Police Plaza this morning, but that didn't mean that
Levitt wouldn't change his mind. Should Jason risk staying to go over the file? If he didn't, he'd have to return
later, not knowing whether Ira would be here or not.
That prospect didn't exactly thrill him. Besides, another
visit to this impenetrable fortress filled with cops and
windows that wouldn't open seemed like too great a risk
to take. And why put off until tomorrow what he could
do today?

❧❧❧

The Slasher case file was a treasure trove of information that had never reached the papers. The NYPD had
slapped a nearly perfect airtight seal on this one. Nothing
was getting out on the investigation that they didn't want
out. The Howard Beach case and the Tawana Brawley fiasco had shown this town's police how dangerous it was
to investigate a crime with the media as your partner.
Fine details of any case with the potentially volatile racial
overtones of this one were now being handled on a de-
partment-wide need-to-know basis. Jason had to agree it
was a smart move, even if it did make his job more difficult.

The files were a revelation. He'd had no idea the victims had been mutilated to this extent. The forensic photos showed headless torsos, severed limbs, and decapitated
heads tossed all over the crime scenes. Each piece had
been hacked, stabbed, and slashed almost beyond recognition.

At two of the scenes, words had been scrawled on the walls in blood—eerie echoes of the Manson family murders. But there was absolutely nothing political or cryptic about these messages. They were loathsome, hate-filled, and brutally basic: "Blood!" "Waste them!" "Kill the Garbage!" "Spicks!" "Cut!" "Die!"

This bloody grafitti was a defiant celebration of the vile crimes that had gained the writer his ink. The erratic sprawling sweep of the letters, like a silent scream, echoed the frenzy with which their author had scrawled them. He would have been splattered with blood by the time he finished his work, unable to walk down a street unnoticed. How had he made his escape? The question taunted Jason.

It taunted the police as well. They'd been searching through all the traffic and parking violations in the areas on the three nights preceding the crimes as well as on the nights of the killings. So far they had turned up nothing, but it had been worth a try; that was how they'd caught Berkowitz.

Reviewing the extensive police files turned up nothing new for Jason—at least nothing tangible in the way of hard facts. But the way Jason saw it, some facts remained immutable—twenty-four dead people; twenty-four reasons why the Slasher should die: Eduardo (age 51), Rosanna (49), Tomás (21), and Jorge Quinoñes (19), Flushing, Queens, May 28; Juan (37), Dolores (34), Julio (14), Marco (13), Pino (12), Hernando (10), Ricardo (8), and Maria Rico (6), Harlem, Manhattan, June 18; Jesús (47), Bonita (32), Luis (13), Carlos (11), Fernando (10), Doris (6), Pedro (5), and Enrique Delmalia (4), Staten Island, June 29; Hernando (44), Maria (40), Laura (17), and José Menguelli (15), Elmhurst, Queens, July 15.

The files, however, did contain the names of several witnesses whom the papers hadn't reported. One in particular caught Jason's interest: Ralph Hunter, a cabdriver, was returning to his Staten Island home around half past midnight on the night of June 29. As he walked from the bus stop he heard what he thought was a woman's scream. The cry ended quickly, so he couldn't tell where it had come from. Two days later he read in the paper about the Delmalia family. They lived only two blocks from his house. He went to the police and reported what he'd heard. The times checked. Ralph had probably heard Bonita Delmalia's final cry. This information confirmed the time of death of the Demalia family but was of no further use to the police. Ralph Hunter hadn't seen anyone on the street and could add no other helpful facts. Maybe that source had dried up for the cops, thought Jason, but it might still hold some possibilities.

Nothing else in the file caught Jason's interest. It was a litany of false leads that went nowhere, interviews that had produced nothing. The Slasher was good at covering his tracks. Or maybe he was just lucky.

❦

His watch showed Jason it was nearly noon. Spending all this time in the very nerve center of a major city's police headquarters was beginning to wear on him; time to get out of there. Vida obviously had the same idea. As he closed his file he saw the FBI agent packing up some notes she'd been jotting down. Jason wished her a good lunch and said he might catch her later. She said good-bye and walked out of the room.

Jason passed Vida in the hall as she stopped to talk to Sergeant Turpin. A short walk down another hall led him to the bank of elevators. As he approached, one of the elevators opened and Ira Levitt stepped out.

Fortunately for Jason, the burly federal agent had his nose buried in a notebook. He walked past Jason without looking up. Jason turned and watched Levitt make his way around the corner to the task force offices. Ira was almost to the door when Vida stepped out.

Jason turned and pressed the elevator call button; the elevator Levitt had come up on had already gone on without him. He could hear Vida and Ira approaching.

"Come on, you mechanical son of a bitch!" he muttered. "Move it!"

For the moment he was out of sight of the two agents, but that was a temporary situation at best. Another two dozen steps on their part would bring him into view. His dyed hair and Vandyke wouldn't fool Levitt.

What the hell was taking the bloody elevators so long? he wondered. Shit! It was lunchtime!

Jason could now hear Levitt and Johnson's conversation as they approached. Why hadn't he thought this through in advance? Because he hadn't. Because he was becoming careless. Because, because, because.

He could imagine people jamming into the elevators, stuffing them full as the lifts stopped at each and every floor.

". . . So I decided to come back here. Guess it's lucky I caught you before you left."

Jason decided to keep his back to Ira and Vida until

they were right on top of him. That way he might be able to take them both down before they could draw their guns.

"Perfect timing. I was on my way out the door," he heard Vida say.

But what if someone else comes along while I'm putting them to sleep? I could end up taking on the whole bloody NYPD!

"Find anything interesting?" Levitt asked.

Why did I come here? It was a stupid, stupid risk!

"No, but I came up with a couple of ideas. I'll tell you about them over lunch. By the way, we're not the only federal agents on this case."

Stupid! Stupid! Stupid!

"The Bureau has someone else here?" Levitt asked.

"No, he's from Justice. As a matter of fact, you must have passed him in the hall."

"What's his name? Maybe I know him."

"Jason Colson. Maybe we'll catch him at the elevator."

But as Ira and Vida turned the corner, all they saw were the doors of a well-stuffed elevator sliding shut.

21

Ralph Hunter was thirty-two, blond, and a little overweight, but even before Jason met him he knew that Hunter's mind would be a pleasure to read. After escaping undetected from Police Plaza Jason had called ahead to let Hunter know that someone from the Justice Department was going to stop by to talk to him regarding the Delmalia case. Ralph's wife had answered the phone and informed Jason that her husband was out, but should be home within the hour. Jason arrived before Ralph's return, so Mrs. Hunter sat him down in their cozy living room and produced a cup of coffee to sip on until her husband returned.

One entire wall of the living room was covered by overflowing bookshelves. While Mrs. Hunter was in the kitchen, Jason took the liberty of checking out the couple's library. There were several Sidney Sheldon and Judith Krantz novels, but there was also a nice selection of Dickens, Shakespeare, Wolfe, Sinclair, and a good many other authors David Vandemark used to enjoy. On the lower shelf was a complete set of Travis McGee novels. MacDonald was one of Jason's favorites, so he figured anyone who liked John D. that much had to have a mind worth looking into.

He was right. Fifteen minutes later Ralph Hunter returned home with two flaxen-haired children in tow. He helped himself to some iced tea from the refrigerator while his daughters began to tear up the house with great glee. The scene rapidly disintegrated into bedlam, whereupon Mrs. Hunter angrily accused her husband of buying the girls ice cream while they were out. Ralph pleaded guilty: double dips. The youngsters' sugar-induced euphoria wasn't going to abate for some time to come, nor could they be induced to go play outside. It was too hot, they said. So Hunter suggested the two men go out to the backyard and talk, leaving Mom to deal with the miniature lunatics he had created.

Once they were settled in a pair of lawn chairs Ralph began to go on about how much he wanted to help the police catch this Slasher. He'd never met the Delmalias, but everyone he'd talked to had said what nice people they'd been. Anything he could do to put that sicko away would be a pleasure. Looking into his mind Jason saw that Ralph was sincere. He also noted, with a grim smile, that the prospect of being involved in a murder case was titillating. Even before meeting Ralph Hunter, Jason had suspected this might be the case. Deep within the middle-class cabbie there lurked an armchair supersleuth.

Jason let Hunter's preamble run its course, then asked the usual investigative questions. Ralph was more than glad to repeat his story about having heard a piercing scream. He said that none of the neighbors had turned on their lights to see what the noise was all about. He supposed they hadn't heard it. After a while Ralph had begun to feel foolish standing there in the dark and had gone home. He hadn't thought about the incident again until he read about the murders in the paper.

Jason telepathically vetted the man's mind as he spoke but turned up nothing new. He hadn't expected to. Not yet. Ralph was telling his story by rote at this point. It had become a monologue he could pull out to astound his friends. Jason needed more information than the standard question-and-answer session would provide.

Ralph ended his tale with "And that's about all I can tell you. I haven't remembered anything new. Sorry."

"Don't be. Your statement confirmed the coroner's estimated time of death for us." Jason knew the police hadn't informed Ralph of this fact and that it would give him a welcome ego boost. He wanted Ralph to feel good before they went any further with the interview.

"Well, that's good to hear," said a smiling Ralph Hunter.

Jason gave Ralph a moment or two to savor his small triumph, then added, "I'd like to do something a touch different with you this time Ralph. I want you to repeat your story to me again, but this time I'd like you to close your eyes and relax when you do it. Take yourself back to the night of June 29. Relive it for me and tell me about it as you go."

"This something like hypnotism?"

"Maybe a bit like self-hypnotism. I'm not going to say a word. Forget I'm here, if you can. Just let your thoughts take you back to that night and experience it all again. Relax."

"Think it would help if I lie on the chaise longue?"

"Let's give it a try and find out."

So Ralph Hunter stretched out on the chaise longue in the shade. "Take all the time you need to get comfortable. We need you in the proper frame of mind, Ralph. I'll just sit here until you're ready."

For the first minute or so Ralph fidgeted, trying to get into the proper mood. Then he settled down and began to focus his thoughts. Jason, who was monitoring them, was pleased at what he felt. Ralph Hunter was going to be an excellent subject. Though whether he'd add any useful information remained to be seen.

All the time Ralph was preparing himself, Jason was doing the same. He wanted to try a deep probe of Ralph Hunter's thoughts, to merge his own consciousness into Ralph Hunter's mind. He'd attempted this only a few times before, with mixed success. Experience had shown him that working with an at-ease, intelligent subject produced the best results. He knew that Hunter had the right ingredients, but there was no telling how the cake would turn out.

In a sleepy voice Ralph Hunter began to talk about getting off the bus and heading home. Boy, was he tired. It had been a long, hot shift. Heavy traffic all afternoon and evening.

Jason felt himself slide into Ralph Hunter's mind. It was like slipping into a groove. Ralph's voice faded. Jason's corporeal self slowly dissolved and was left behind. It was like an out-of-body experience, except that he was inside the taxi driver's mind. It was the best connection he'd ever made. Jason found himself walking down the dimly lit Staten Island street. He was actually *there*, just as much as Ralph was, and the man was doing a bang-up job of reliving the experience.

Ralph Hunter's mental images were as sharp as any Jason had ever experienced. A foggy haze hovered around the edges, but the center of each mental image was crystal clear. Even details that Ralph couldn't consciously recall were there. Jason had managed to link up with the man's subconscious. He could barely suppress his elation. Jason had managed to successfully link with a person's subconscious only twice before, and never this strongly.

Jason and Ralph walked down the street together. They pulled out a stick of gum, popped it into their mouth, tossed the wrapper away. Most of the houses around them were dark. Occasionally they saw a light in a window. This was a working-class neighborhood. Early to bed, early to rise. Two cats raced down a driveway, ran across the street, and disappeared into the shadows. The sedans and station wagons, parked bumper to bumper along the street, were empty. At the end of the block Jason and Ralph spit out their gum. It was still too hot for anything that sweet.

They moved onto the next block. Jason noticed a large yellow Ryder rental truck parked on the far side of the street, which Ralph's conscious mind hadn't registered. It was empty. Probably someone planning to move the next day. Fewer lights shone in the windows on this block. There weren't even any pets around.

This was where the murders had occurred.

The scream tore out of the darkness. It was more of a shriek than a scream, actually, like the nocturnal cry of a large bird of prey. It ended abruptly after lasting a much shorter time than Ralph consciously remembered. Less than a second. The abrupt end was unnerving. Their fight-or-flight impulses flooded with adrenaline, Ralph and Jason's pulse immediately went into high gear. They stood there, vainly trying to determine where the sound had come from. No luck. They retraced their steps back a couple of houses. Still nothing. The two of them surveyed the darkened houses. No lights here at all.

Jason could sense the confusion in Ralph's thoughts. What should he do? What had he really heard? It was a scream, but what did it mean? Maybe someone was having a fight. Or perhaps someone had burned herself taking a teapot off the stove. Preparing tea in the dark? Maybe the kitchen was at the back of the house, where he couldn't see the light. Hell, the scream could have come from the next street over. It was probably nothing. He should forget about it and go home.

Near the end of the block Jason took note of another vehicle that Ralph hadn't paid any conscious attention to—a tan commercial van. There was lettering on the side of it, but the van wasn't near a streetlight, so Jason couldn't read the logo.

They crossed over to the next block. Only two lights on in this stretch. Halfway down the block Jason and Ralph spotted a young couple sitting on a darkened porch, huddled together, speaking softly. Had they heard the scream? Probably not. They were nearly a block away. Jason wondered why this couple hadn't been mentioned in Ralph's statement. But the reason became clear almost immediately. They couldn't have been involved in the killings. They were young lovers stealing a few precious moments together on the front porch. The girl's parents most likely didn't even know she was out here. Why get her into trouble? Ralph had been young once.

The last half block to Ralph's house held nothing of interest, but Jason heard a car engine start farther up the block. No way to check it out, though, because Ralph hadn't noticed it. Living in a heavily populated area gave one a knack for turning off sounds one didn't want to hear.

Jason broke off contact and let Ralph finish his reminiscing. He had cleared away the cobwebs by the time Hunter opened his eyes and asked, "Well? How'd I do?"

"Just fine, Ralph. There's a couple points you brought up I think I'll check on."

"Like what?"

"I'd rather not say anything right now. But if I turn anything up, I might want to talk to you again. Thanks."

They shook hands, and Jason departed, leaving Ralph Hunter feeling that he was involved in something really important, though he couldn't be sure exactly what it was.

Jason slowly backtracked down the street he had just traveled with Hunter, the bright sunlight playing through the canopy of trees.

He stopped where he remembered the Ryder truck being parked. Looking around, he spotted a house with a For Sale sign on the front lawn. Jason confirmed that it was indeed empty. Well, that explained the rental truck.

Next, Jason doubled back to where the tan van had been. He started knocking on doors, showing his credentials and asking questions. Nobody knew of anyone in the area who owned such a vehicle. Several people told Jason that Herb Jackson, down the street, had a green van. But no one remembered a tan one.

So what did that give him? A car starting up the street

from Ralph's house and a tan van that didn't belong to anyone in the neighborhood. Not much.

Jason decided he could write off the car up the street. What did the killer do? Slash his victims, then jump out a rear window, race down to the next street over, hurriedly get a half block ahead of Ralph, jump into his waiting car, and start it up as Hunter reached his door? Not likely. The starting car didn't mean anything. It was a red herring.

The tan van, on the other hand, might be a real lead. But what kind? He hadn't been able to read what it said on the side of the vehicle. Hadn't even gotten a glimpse of the license plate. There had to be several hundred tan vans driving around the Greater New York area. So the odds of finding this vehicle were slim to none.

Jason walked back to Victory Boulevard, hailed a cab, and hunkered down in the backseat to brood. It looked like this trip to scenic Staten Island had been a monumental waste, and so was this mental funk, he realized. He spent the rest of the cab ride going over everything he had experienced in his union with Ralph Hunter. Maybe he'd missed something the first time around. But by the time the cab reached the ferry station Jason could see he'd thoroughly exhausted that avenue of investigation. In his boredom he was beginning to mentally add werewolves and vampires to his midnight stroll with Mr. Hunter.

The ride back to Manhattan on the ferry gave Jason a chance to sort his thoughts and put them in their proper perspective. This cheered him and convinced him that he was better off than he would have admitted twenty minutes ago. The police files had given him a much clearer picture of how the Slasher operated. Also, his walk down the street on the night of the killings had revealed that the killer was human. He had screwed up. One of his victims had survived long enough to scream. That foul-up could cost the Slasher his freedom. He'd made one mistake already. He would make others.

But the most important result of this day's labors was learning that Ira Levitt was in town looking for him. Jason knew he'd have to remain alert to avoid bumping into his pursuer again. That episode at the elevators was something he never wanted to repeat.

Yes, Jason was a bit farther along in the hunt than he had been this morning. He still didn't know the Slasher's identity, but he was a few steps closer to uncovering that secret.

A cab ride uptown returned Jason to his van, where he changed into Leroy De Carlo's clothes and identity. When he finished his transformation, Leroy glanced at his watch and hissed, "Damn!"

It was 6:45 P.M. He was late for his dinner date with Angela. My, how time did fly when you were on the scent.

22

Charles Camden pressed one of the numerous buttons on the inset console atop his otherwise bare desk. A panel in the center retracted and an IBM PC rose to take the console's place. He pulled a floppy disk from a desk drawer and slipped it into the internal drive.

The two men standing nearby had watched this procedure before. They were hard men, not easily awed, but the man at the computer was someone they respected and feared. They'd worked for him for years and were well aware of the power he wielded. That was why neither spoke, nor would they, until Charles Camden addressed them first.

Camden called up a file, and a list of names appeared on the screen. He scrolled through it, searching. As the names crawled by he noted that four of them were marked with an asterisk and eight others with an X.

The four names with asterisks were Eduardo Quiñoñes, Juan Rico, Jesús Delmalia, and Hernando Menguelli; the eight marked X meant that these persons had either moved or were for some other reason unsuitable for Charles Camden's needs.

All the names had a number of things in common. Every one of them was at one time on welfare. Camden had found these candidates by accessing the Welfare Department's data base, which provided a wealth of personal information on clients: names and ages of all family members, addresses, work history, and general background.

Membership in this club also meant these men and women were poor. That was important to Camden. It meant no one would raise a hue and cry over their death—at least not the kind of hue and cry that meant anything. The newspapers would sensationalize the murders, but no one would give a shit if a bunch of welfare deadbeats got their tickets punched. Being poor meant they were stuck in the crosshairs, within the boundaries of the sociological strata Camden was targeting.

Every name on the list was Hispanic—the most important commonality, as far as Camden was concerned—and everyone on the list lived in New York.

Everyone on the list was the head of a family of at least four.

So all of them were potential victims of the Latino Family Killer.

So many victims, so little time. Finally Charles Camden selected two names. Alfredo Martinez, who lived in the Bronx, and Esteban Moreno of Brooklyn.

Camden typed a few more commands into the computer and sat back to survey the results. A concealed printer on the lower left side of his desk sprang to life. When it fell silent, Charles Camden tore off the two printouts and handed one to each of the waiting men. "Here you go."

"Same procedure?" one of them asked.

"Yes, everything you can come up with," Camden answered.

The two men nodded in unison, turned in tandem, and left the office. Camden knew they'd get the job done without any questions. The two of them had been with him since Vietnam. They'd learned a long time ago that it was best not to know everything their boss was up to. Both of them had known other Company operatives who'd gotten too nosy. Camden's boys were still here. The inquisitive ones weren't. Neither knew where the others had gone. Neither cared to know. These were good men. They knew how to follow orders.

"Alfredo Martinez. Esteban Moreno." In the tranquil solitude of his office Charles Camden spoke the names softly, almost as if praying. And that was the way it should be, he thought. One must always speak reverently of the dead and the soon to be so.

23

Leroy was delighted to find that Angela had not been waiting impatiently for him, drumming her fingernails on a table. She had taken the opportunity to change clothes. The light print dress she looked so good in that morning had been replaced by a modest dark blue suit. The garb was much more appropriate for the task at hand: visiting a woman who had lost her entire family only four weeks ago. He applauded her foresight while remembering it had been only seven weeks since Angela had lost her own family. He was struck once more by her strength, her remarkable spirit.

Leroy knew that during dinner—at an Italian restaurant two blocks from the apartment—the conversation would likely move toward an exchange of personal histories. He was prepared for this. Being a highly experienced liar, Leroy had no trouble presenting an edited version of David Vandemark's life story, so far as he remembered it. He and Angela exchanged childhood reminiscences and discovered they had much in common. Both of them had been the odd person out during their high-school years, too introverted to be popular. All that had changed.

They were like any other couple dining out and getting to know each other. Forgotten for the moment was the Slasher haunting New York City. It was as if Leroy De Carlo had no other purpose in life than to enjoy this beautiful lady's company. Gone were the tragic circumstances that had brought this strange man into Angela Quinoñes's world. Good food and conversation—what need was there for anything else?

Everything went beautifully until Angela asked Leroy why he'd given up law to become a private investigator. He'd planned to give her a song and dance about getting bored with the work and wanting some excitement. Angela would have bought that story, and it would have kept things from getting complicated, but instead, Leroy found himself telling her how he had once been married to a wonderful woman named Christine. He also spoke about his daughter. He couldn't stop himself. The story seemed to tell itself. An accident had laid him up in the hospital, he said. While he was there, his wife and child were killed by a madman, a serial killer. When he got back on his feet, he hunted down the murderer. Leroy neglected to mention that he was able to do this with the aid of telepathic powers and that he'd pumped two .38 caliber slugs into Greg Hewett upon catching up with him. After that he'd realized he couldn't return to his old life. Leroy said quite sincerely that he found his new career much more satisfying than the law had ever been.

When he finished, Leroy fell silent, lost in thoughts all his own. Angela assumed he was remembering his beloved wife and child, and she sat quietly, waiting for

Leroy to return to the present. But Leroy was wondering why he had told Angela about Chris and Jennifer. It wasn't the story that bothered him. It was the way it had made him feel.

Leroy De Carlo, the man with many names, who had risen out of the ashes of David Vandemark, had spoken of Chris and Jenny's death as his personal loss. But why? He wasn't David Vandemark! The only thing he and Vandemark had in common was the body they each inhabited at different times. But it was true. There was no denying it. Leroy had felt a deep personal loss as he told of the murders. He didn't get it. Those people meant nothing to him. What was going on inside his head?

Angela's words came to him as if across a vast distance. "Are you all right, Leroy?"

He snapped out of it, faced her, and smiled weakly. "Yes . . . yes. Guess I was wool-gathering. Sorry. I don't talk about Chris and Jenny too often."

"It's not good to keep those things bottled up inside. That was one of the first things I decided after I lost my family. It wouldn't be right never to speak of them. Sure, it was painful. But they'd been part of my life. Not thinking or talking about them would be like denying they ever existed. And I think they deserve better."

"I guess talking probably helps the healing process along."

"Yes, I think so. I'm sure it's helped me."

Leroy reached across the table and squeezed Angela's hand. "You know, you're really quite a lady. I think you've handled your family tragedy better in seven weeks than I have in seven years."

As Leroy was about to pull his hand back Angela gently squeezed it and looked into his eyes with a startling directness. "I've got a good ear, De Carlo, if you ever need it." Calling him De Carlo gave her the courage to keep holding on to his hand. "Remember, I owe you for what you're doing to hunt down that animal."

Leroy felt himself flush. All he could say was "Thanks. I'll keep that in mind."

Angela gave his hand another squeeze and released it. Leroy was sorry to have the contact end. But it was for the best. "I better get the bill," he said. "We ought to be heading uptown."

∞∞∞∞

The neighborhood where Mrs. Vallejo lived wasn't nearly as bad as Leroy had imagined. He had read, of course, that certain sections of Spanish Harlem were experiencing urban renewal. And here was living proof. Though this would not have been mistaken for an upscale neighborhood, there was no longer the overriding tension in the air that he'd noticed while visiting the area on a previous hunt.

Stoops were crowded with people—a mix of blacks and Hispanics—hanging out, seeking relief from the heat. The air was filled with sounds of salsa, hip-hop, and Latino pop. An old man sat under a streetlight, across from a bodega, reading *El Diario*. Kids had gathered on street corners, laughing and chattering in a strange mixture of English and Spanish. For a moment Leroy's midwestern brain felt magically transported to some exotic foreign land. Then the reality check of New York's grimy streets turned his sensory prism a notch and everything fell into place. The street sign at 112th and Broadway underscored the point.

No one seemed to notice when Angela and Leroy got out of the cab. Angela's natural coloring and his own recently manufactured Latin look allowed them to fit in unnoticed.

A question tugged at Leroy's mind: Why had the Slasher chosen such a crowded urban area? The chances of being spotted must have been phenomenal. Even at one in the morning, when the Rico family had been murdered, there had to have been people on the street. Why take the risk? Or was the risk factor somehow the key? Was this the Slasher's way of saying something? What was his message? That no matter where you live, if you're Hispanic, you're not safe?

∽∾∾∾

Rosita Vallejo, age forty-two, was dressed in black and spoke in a whisper. She was a small woman, the kind who, if animated, would have reminded Leroy of a bright, glittering-eyed bird, but this loss had taken all the spirit out of her. There was a terrible emptiness in her eyes that touched even Leroy's callous heart. The third-floor three-bedroom walk-up seemed positively cavernous as they passed through it to the living room, oddly situated at the back of the apartment. Leroy could faintly perceive, on some preternatural level, the violence these walls had witnessed. He could not sense enough to attempt any kind of reading, but he knew that ghosts still walked these rooms. On the living-room wall hung a family portrait draped in black silk.

Angela explained why she and Leroy were there. Mrs. Vallejo was encouraged to hear that someone from the outside had been brought in to investigate the killings. She didn't have much faith in the New York police. They had made her grief sound like yesterday's news. Yes, of course, she'd be happy to help Señor De Carlo in any way that she could. It was the only time during the entire visit that Leroy saw life flicker briefly in her eyes.

With Angela as his interpreter, Leroy learned that Mrs. Vallejo had come to New York from Puerto Rico after her husband died in an auto accident a year ago. Her brother, Juan, had sent her plane fare and found her a job with a downtown office-cleaning service. Rosita worked from midnight to eight.

She would be moving out of the apartment soon. It was too large and held too many memories. Besides, she didn't earn nearly enough to pay the rent. It wouldn't be easy finding a studio, with rents so high. From her mind Leroy gleaned her worry that she would find herself one of those poor old women who haunt Manhattan's streets, carrying their worldly possessions in shopping bags.

Through Angela, Leroy asked Rosita to tell him about the night of the killings. Slowly, hesitantly, she began her story. She told it a few sentences at a time, giving Angela plenty of time to translate.

"She says that at about eleven-thirty a co-worker stopped by, as usual, to walk her to the subway. Most of the family was in bed, but Juan was still up, watching the news. He asked Rosita to pick up a quart of milk on her way home. Everything seemed normal. There was no way of knowing the terrible scene she would find when she returned.

"Her shift at work went smoothly, and she started home at seven-thirty. She doesn't have to punch a time clock; when the work's finished, she goes home.

"She stopped at a bodega for a quart of milk and went home. Other people were starting their day as Rosita was ending hers. She said hello to a few neighbors as she made her way up to the apartment. Juan's wife, Dolores, had a job, so the place was deserted during the day. She usually slept until the kids returned from school around three-thirty.

"As soon as she entered the apartment she knew something terrible had happened. There was blood on the walls. Blood on the floor. Words written in blood. Blood everywhere. All the bedroom doors were open. She walked to the nearest one, the boys' room."

Rosita Vallejo couldn't go on. She sobbed uncontrollably into her hands. Angela offered the distraught woman a tissue.

Leroy got to his feet. "Tell her she doesn't have to describe what she found here. I already got that from the police reports. See if you can calm her down."

Angela wrapped an arm around Mrs. Vallejo's shoulders as Leroy wandered out of the room and down the pristine hallway to the kitchen. He wondered who had cleaned the walls after the police had finished their investigation. Surely not the police. Rosita? Her friend from work? He hoped it hadn't been Rosita.

Leroy searched through the kitchen cabinets until he found what he was after. He tossed a splash of rum into a glass, returned to the living room, and gave it to Mrs. Vallejo. She accepted it without fuss and sipped on it as she composed herself.

When she had recovered enough to continue, Leroy instructed Angela to ask her about the life of the Rico family both before and after she came to live with them.

For the next half hour Rosita spoke of her family, a family that struggled hard to survive in an unforgiving city. Juan worked for the transit system. He made good money, but it wasn't enough to support a large family. So five years ago, shortly after the youngest child was born, Dolores Rico had gotten herself a job as a secretary. A neighbor kept an eye on the kids. They were good children. No trouble. No trouble at all.

Rosita told how kind the family had been taking her in last year. Unable to speak the language, Rosita knew she was a burden to them, but they never complained. She was family. Relatives didn't desert one another. Rosita tried to repay their kindness by taking a job as quickly as possible. She didn't like her work, but she was glad to help ease the financial burden on the family.

Leroy listened intently to her entire tale, trying to find something that would connect the Rico family to the other victims. Rosita continued her narrative by relating what she knew about the family's life before her arrival.

Juan had come to the States in the early eighties. He and Dolores met, fell in love, and were married. Their first years of marriage were tough. Juan was going to night school and working during the day. Dolores became pregnant with their first child, Julio, just about the time the gas station where Juan worked went out of business. Rosita remembered Juan saying what a hard time that was for them. His unemployment insurance had run out and they were forced to apply for welfare. Luckily he soon got a job with the MTA, and things had been fairly good since then. Tight, but manageable.

Leroy and Angela exchanged glances at the mention of welfare.

When Rosita ran out of things to remember, Angela thought that would end the interview. But it didn't, and she was surprised by what Leroy asked Mrs. Vallejo to do next. He repeated the directions he'd given Ralph Hunter earlier in the day, and Angela translated the request. "Mrs. Vallejo, could you relax, please, and close your eyes? We want you to let your mind take you back to when you and your friend left the apartment and headed to work on the night of the murders. Relive the moment and tell us everything you see."

Angela had never seen a detective on television use this technique. But De Carlo was a professional and presumably knew what he was doing. Mrs. Vallejo agreed to give it a try. She sat back in her chair and tried to get comfortable. Leroy closed his eyes soon after Mrs. Vallejo did.

While listening to Mrs. Vallejo's story Leroy had been monitoring her thoughts. Past experience had shown him that scanning the mind of a non-English-speaking subject wasn't that different from tapping someone who did speak the language. Most telepathic communication consisted of picture images and auditory sensations with some olfactory memories, overlaid with emotions. Some words were mixed in there, but far fewer than one would imagine. Leroy lost a small part of the message because of the language barrier, but he got ninety percent of it. While Mrs. Vallejo had been speaking Leroy had acclimated himself to her thought processes and mental rhythms, getting in tune with her.

He knew Rosita Vallejo wouldn't be the model subject for a deep probe that Ralph Hunter had been. She was too distracted by her own grief to relax totally, especially with two strangers sitting nearby. But maybe he could pick up something.

At last Mrs. Vallejo seemed relaxed and ready to begin. With her eyes shut and her pinched features beginning to soften, she began to tell how she had left the apartment.

For Leroy, the connection was bad. It was blurry, jumpy, fading in and out as Mrs. Vallejo's concentration waxed and waned. Leroy feared that he was wasting his time. In the distance he could hear the woman talking and Angela translating, but the words were indistinguishable. Mrs. Vallejo's train of thought was nearly as jumbled. There was no subconscious contact this time.

❧❧❧❧

Leroy and Mrs. Vallejo were walking down the stairs of the apartment building with her co-worker, Bernard Cowan. He was talking about something, but Rosita wasn't listening. She was thinking about the long night of work that lay ahead.

Then everything got blurry and seemed to rush ahead like a videotape on fast-forward. Leroy could vaguely see Mrs. Vallejo's feet as she watched her step going down the stairs. He could hear the sound of her breathing, but Bernard Cowan's voice faded into a static hum.

The picture focused when they reached the second-floor landing. Leroy and Mrs. Vallejo said hello to Mrs.

Vasquez, a terrible gossip who lived two floors below the Vallejo apartment.

The rest of the trip down the stairs was mostly a blur—nothing Mrs. Vallejo considered important enough to remember. Only when they reached the building's front door did she refocus her attention on Cowan, as he held it open for Rosita. This gave Leroy his first clear look at Cowan, a large, good-looking black man in his mid-forties, neatly dressed, and clearly enjoying Rosita's company.

Out on the street, Mrs. Vallejo saw a young couple she knew; Leroy didn't catch their names. Then the visual images started to flicker. Rosita hadn't paid much attention to her surroundings. Why should she? It was the same street she'd walked hundreds of times. Damn! This wasn't going to do Leroy any good. How was he going to find a clue to the Slasher's identity when his eyewitness hadn't bothered to look at her surroundings on the night of the murder?

The images kept jumping in and out of focus as Leroy and his two traveling companions made their way down the block. He could make out the blurred shapes of people walking past and cars parked along the street. But everything was out of focus, with little or no detail. Leroy was about to give up, when a large beige shape approached.

To Leroy's surprise, the beige shape sprang into focus. With a start, he realized the shape wasn't beige. It was tan! And it was a van! The lettering on the side of the vehicle was crystal clear this time.

"You saw a van, didn't you?" Leroy nearly shouted as he sat upright.

Angela and Mrs. Vallejo were staring at him as if he had lost his mind. "She just said that. Does that mean something?"

"Ask her what color it was."

Angela did so and replied, "Light brown. Very light. I guess that means tan."

"Why did she notice it?"

Again Angela translated, got her answer, and said, "This building has a problem with roaches. The van belonged to an exterminating company, and Rosita was going to talk to her brother about calling them."

An exterminator. Talk about your black humor. Leroy closed his eyes and saw the tan van with the crisp black lettering on its passenger door, very businesslike: Taglia Exterminators. There was a phone number underneath it. He immediately consigned the name and number to memory.

Thirty minutes later, after administering one more medicinal dose of rum, Leroy and Angela made their way down the tenement stairs. Leroy, deep in thought, absentmindedly ran his hand along the railing. As they neared the bottom landing Angela couldn't stand the suspense any longer. "The extermination van. You got an important clue there, didn't you?"

"Maybe. There was a vehicle like it parked in the neighborhood on the night of the Delmalia murders. The person who noticed it didn't remember the name on its side. It's worth—"

Leroy was about to step off the stairs when he froze, his eyes wide and staring into the void. Angela turned around on the landing below him. "It's worth what?" she asked.

The expression on Leroy's face, one of shock and confusion, turned icy. Angela watched his gaze travel to his hand, gripping the railing with white-knuckled intensity.

Somehow, despite all the people who'd traipsed over the crime scene, this one small section of the railing had not been touched, disturbed, or contaminated. The odds against Leroy finding it were a million to one. But the impression was unmistakable and startling.

The man stood in the dark, his eyes struggling to pierce the shadowed recesses of the upper stairwell, occasionally darting toward the street.

He was frightened, terrified, barely holding on to his composure, hanging in there only because he was a pro.

Leroy tried to focus on the man but found his features frustratingly elusive. There was too much emotion in play. Fear and rising panic. Not enough conscious, rational thought.

The man was scared of what he was doing, of what was going on upstairs. Of being caught. But that fear was kept in check by something evil. Something very civilized and powerful. Someone to be feared even more than the monster three flights up.

Leroy spoke the name of the object of this man's fear.

"Camden."

24

The first half of the taxi ride home passed wordlessly. Leroy and Angela were entertaining their own thoughts. Rosita's story had gotten more than a few wheels turning. The neon glow of the city slipped past unnoticed. Angela turned abruptly and asked, "So what's with the welfare angle? You think the Slasher's killing families that have been on welfare?"

"Or were on it when they were killed, like the Delmalia family. Jesús Delmalia lost an arm in an industrial accident six months ago. They'd been on the welfare rolls for two months. I'm sure I'll find that the Menguellis were on public assistance at one time as well."

"The Slasher is killing welfare families? But why?"

"I won't find that out until I get my hands on him, I'm afraid. Even then his reasons may not be anything you or I would understand."

"Maybe our killer is Newt Gingrich," muttered Angela as she gazed at Leroy, trying to read him. "What was it you started to tell me on the stairs?"

"Something came to me. I'm not sure what it means yet."

There was nothing more to be read in Leroy's features; he was too good a poker player. She decided not to press the matter, but she didn't take her eyes off her uncommunicative traveling companion. This mystery man was terribly attractive, she told herself. His jet-black Vandyke made him look very dashing.

⊷∾∾⊷

When the cab dropped them off at Angela's apartment she walked directly up to the front door. After unlocking it, she noticed Leroy hadn't followed her up the stoop.

"Think I'll be heading off to find myself a hotel room," he said.

Without stopping to think, Angela stepped down to him and reached for his hand. "Don't." It sounded like both a plea and a command. Her eyes, when he looked at them, were huge and luminous.

Leroy knew he couldn't leave now. He was caught in those eyes, swimming in their twin pools. Trapped like a bug in amber. He threw any niggling sense of misgiving, together with caution, to the winds.

Angela led him up four flights of steps in silence. Only when she had closed the apartment door behind them did she speak. "Don't leave me alone tonight. There's been too much death. I . . . I couldn't . . ."

She lifted her face to him. Without realizing he'd made the decision to do so, Leroy kissed her. It was a gentle and lingering kiss. Soft lips, moist, slightly parted. He gently drew her to him and felt her arms slip smoothly around his neck. The heat of the kiss intensified. A moment became eternity.

When they pulled away, he was gasping for air like a
man drowning, his lungs burning. But it was an effort that
brought no relief. Angela buried her face in his neck,
kissing it and rubbing her cheek against it. He found an
earlobe and felt her breath quicken. Their mouths found
each other again. Her tongue probed deep into his
mouth.

Then he was lifting her into his arms, their lips insepa-
rable. Leroy's tongue was exploring her mouth. He was
vaguely aware of walking toward the bedroom. Everything seemed to be happening in slow motion or under
water; he wasn't sure which. Something was happening to
his sense of time, too. And there were whole sections of
their journey across the apartment on which Leroy drew a
blank. He couldn't remember how he had maneuvered
through this doorway or avoided tripping over that piece
of furniture. Things were fragmenting. Falling to pieces.
But it all felt so goddamn good, who the hell cared?

The next thing he knew they were in Angela's bed,
nuzzling and stroking each other. Clothes were shed
slowly as they kissed and caressed every patch of bare
flesh they could find on one another. There was no awkwardness to it. It was like a dance. And their choreogra-
phy would have made Twyla Tharp jealous. Leroy could
feel his self slipping away. He was becoming part of the
one, merging with this beautiful woman, joining more
than just their bodies. Magic!

Fragmentation . . .

Leroy kissed and ran his tongue along her neck, shoulders, and breasts. Finding her nipples, he sucked gently
on them, feeling them harden in his mouth. Her moans
of pleasure were like music. Yet not even Schubert ever

penned such a marvelously sweet melody. His heart felt as if it might burst from his chest. The room filled with an effluvium, a fragrant musk, a torrid urgency. Hot. Desperate. Mad.

Fragmentation . . .

They were on their knees now in the center of the bed, their bodies pressed together, moving rhythmically. Leroy could feel her hands stroking and caressing him, driving him to the sweetest sort of insanity. It was all just too good! He couldn't take much more of this without dying or bursting into flames, his head blowing off his shoulders like Krakatoa. Dying of pleasure. Crazy! Had to stop it. Couldn't.

Fragmentation . . .

His own hands trailed softly up and down her back, eliciting small groans of delight. She clasped him between her thighs, working a rhythm older than time immemorial, a rhythm that played in both their heads.

Fragmentation . . .

Lying on their sides now, no idea how they got there. His hand between her thighs, gently stroking her. Angela's back arched in sudden explosive release. Her cry echoed through the dimly lit room, loud and throaty. Strange that joy often sounded so much like mayhem. Everything so much like a dream.

Fragmentation . . .

He kissed her stomach, lost amid the myriad pleasures that were Angela, his face buried in her soft fur, his tongue working. Once again she exploded beneath him. Once again he was lost in her pleasure.

Fragmentation . . .

Now linked, grasping, gasping, trying to pull each other

closer together. Beneath them the sheets tangled and un-
tangled as their frantic dance continued unabated and
seemingly without end, rising to heights undreamed of.
Linked and traveling through the universe with the most
ravishing creature he had ever known. Lost in her beauty,
her grace, her strength.

Fragmentation . . .

The entire universe exploded in a mad kaleidoscopic
frenzy, as if lightning had struck. And everything else was
swept away in a blinding flash. They clung desperately to
each other as the world ended in fire.

Spent, limbs tangled, drenched in joyous sweat, they
continued to kiss, still lost in each other. Exhausted, drifting off, a single thought stirred in David Vandemark's
mind. It was beautiful. Heaven. No need to tell her. She
knew as well as he did, but she didn't know why. Why
was it so different? Because it was the first time in over
seven years that he'd made love to anybody he really
cared about. David triumphantly carried that thought
with him into the realm of Morpheus.

❦

Rolling over in her sleep, Angela woke David. He
stared uncomprehendingly at his surroundings, which
were dimly illuminated by light from another room.

Where was he? He didn't know, but he felt great.

Then it came back to him, and he looked tenderly at
the beautiful woman beside him. A small kiss on her ear
was rewarded with a satisfied sleepy purr. After that the
only sound in the room was her even breathing.

David gently pulled the tangled sheet up over Angela's

shoulder and carefully got out of the bed. David did, not Leroy. It was David who dug his cigarettes out of his crumpled sport coat. Not bothering to dress, he stepped naked into the living room and turned off the light.

Perched on the arm of the sofa, David found himself shivering as he communed with the night. Yes, he was David Vandemark. Always had been. The masquerade was over. And a symbolic domino mask lay among his things on the floor of the bedroom. A barrier had been demolished. The lady had shattered it with a kiss. Things could never be the same again. The illusion that he and David Vandemark were two different people was gone forever. She had touched something within him that he had believed was dead.

Without warning, the past swept over David like a tidal wave, and suddenly he remembered the terrifying maelstrom that was his return to consciousness in that hospital bed in Detroit.

25

Voices come out of the all-encompassing darkness. Words from the void. Voices overlapping and intertwining, creating an indecipherable din. An overwhelming racket. Babel. Terrifying.

After about a million years of torment, the chaos subsides. And all but one of the voices fade into the pitch-black distance. Then it hits you. A chilling realization. One that makes no sense. Those aren't voices you are hearing. They are something else.

The remaining voice drones on. You listen, trying to understand exactly what this is you're experiencing. That is the only word that fits. *Experiencing*. You're not hearing the voice, you're . . .

Its garbled message washes over you in gentle waves. This you can tolerate, even though you don't understand it. Clarity occurs slowly. This is definitely something new. Something incomprehensible. The unique voice speaks, but not in words. Some words are mixed into the message, but there are also visual images, audio and tactile sensations. This can't be real. It's got to be some kind of dream.

But it doesn't feel like a dream.

If it is a dream, then there is one sure way to end it. And ending it seems like a great idea. It's too creepy. Too weird. Wake up and get out of this unsettling fantasy! You don't want to be here! Wake up! You can do it! You can . . .

Pain!

It cuts you like a hot knife! You must get away from it! Back off! Run!

It's subsiding rapidly. You can relax now. You retreated from it. Crept farther back into the void, where it's safe.

But you can't feel pain in your dreams. That agony was real. Your ribs and leg ached horribly. And your head felt as if it had been cracked open and set afire. You'd never before felt the sheer power and majesty of such intolerable pain. Bottomless and totally endless, like the universe itself.

And it didn't feel like a dream.

So what now? Do you lie here and wonder? No. If you're not mad already, you soon will be if you do nothing. You must find out what's going on. You don't want to feel that pain again, but how else can you discover whether you're dreaming? And if you aren't dreaming, then how can you be sure your current state won't last forever?

Who was it that claimed he'd prefer an eternity of pain over a lifetime of feeling nothing? Smart man.

But there has to be a way around the pain. Some other method to determine if you're sleeping.

Time!

That's the answer! When you're sleeping, time doesn't

mean anything. You've got no sense of it. Time passes unnoticed.

Count to sixty, slowly. Make the count clear and precise. Don't let your mind wander. Focus all your attention on it.

1, 2, 3, 4, 5, 6, 7, 8, 9, 10, 11, 12, 13, 14, 15, 16, 17, 18, 19, 20, 21, 22, 23, 24, 25, 26, 27, 28, 29, 30, 31, 32, 33, 34, 35, 36, 37, 38, 39, 40, 41, 42, 43, 44, 45, 46, 47, 48, 49, 50, 51, 52, 53, 54, 55, 56, 57, 58, 59, 60.

You did it! Now do it again.

And again.

Do it ten times!

Ten times. Ten minutes. This is no dream. You're not sleeping. Don't you remember reading that rapid-eye-movement sleep lasts for only ninety seconds to two minutes? You dream during REM sleep and only then. You counted out ten minutes. You're not dreaming. You're not sleeping.

Then what *are* you doing?

You're in some type of conscious state, even though you don't appear to be conscious. But you are aware, like someone in a kind of deep trance. How did you come to be in this condition?

You're not asleep, but you're not fully awake, either.

You must wake up. That's the only way to solve this mystery.

But the pain . . .

You've got to face it. Somehow you'll find the strength. You must. It's either pain or the distinct possibility of spending an eternity in limbo. Which is it going to be?

You steel yourself. The pain isn't quite so devastating this time. Sure, it runs over you, kicks you around, stomps you flat, and then bites you on the ass for good measure. But finally it subsides, though not completely. It just lowers the volume to a nearly tolerable level. And then memory returns.

You remember the elevator. The crash. Are you still lying at the bottom of that shaft? No, you must have been rescued by now.

Try to move. See if you can feel a bed or twisted metal beneath you. Maybe you can't pierce this black veil that clouds your vision, but you can feel. You can . . . you . . . you . . .

You can't do that, either. Can't move! You don't feel anything!

Panic!

Paralyzed!

You can't lift a finger or raise an eyelid. You're trapped inside a body that's unable to move.

Remember that book you read back in college? *Johnny Got His Gun*. Oh, God. About a World War I soldier who loses his face, ears, and limbs. The wretched bastard spends the rest of his days hallucinating horrors. Is that to be your fate? No! You will not believe that! Not you.

Medical science has come so far since then. Those damn doctors could keep you imprisoned in this motionless flesh, balancing on the precipice between life and death, for another fifty, sixty years.

You wail in fear and loathing, a scream that does not pass your lips but echoes and re-echoes throughout the black void for several millennia.

It takes that long for you to come to terms with this horrible possibility. But then, humans are remarkably resilient creatures, capable of adjusting to the cruelest of fates. Especially when they have no choice. After all, ending your suffering by suicide is hardly an option when you can't raise your hands to slip the noose around your neck.

The hysteria fades. You sit alone within the void. Helpless. And oh, so lonely.

But not for long. The voices return. Thank God! At least now they'll keep you company.

There's no telling how long it takes you to learn how to focus on a single voice. They usually come in groups, a deluge of chaotic messages, sensory overload. But you slowly learn how to control the sounds. You teach yourself to screen out the unwanted ones. You silence them with your will so that you can be surrounded by dozens of the voices and hear only one. You zero in on that one, embrace it, and the others fade from your consciousness.

Until now some part of your rational mind has suspected that the visual images and the accompanying sensations are hallucinatory. But that's not so, is it? Time has confirmed their reality. They are as real as anything else you're experiencing. Which leaves only one explanation. Holmes once told Watson that after you eliminate the impossible what remains, no matter how improbable, is the truth. Reality.

David Vandemark, your truth is telepathy. You're reading minds.

That's how you learn of the extent of your injuries. Your spirits soar. From the minds of visiting doctors and nurses you learn that you are not paralyzed. You have been in a coma for almost three days, but your prognosis is good. You have a strong pulse and excellent respiration. They expect you to regain consciousness at any time.

The only fear you see within their thoughts is of that faceless demon, brain damage. You wish you could speak to them, tell them that your brain is running with the precision of a fine Swiss watch. It's the rest of you that's not operational.

From their minds you gain a clearer sense of time.

That is how you know that it's the following day when you begin to bridge the gap between mind and body. You feel crisp sheets and a soft mattress beneath you.

Control over motor skills begins to return slowly; it takes most of a day for you to twitch a little toe and finger. It's difficult, requiring intense concentration. When the voices are present, they distract you, make it impossible to display your progress. So the concerned voices never suspect the rapid recovery taking place within the inert form. Only you know the darkness is lifting.

A nurse comes to check your vital signs. As you monitor her mind, you pick up some frightening thoughts.

A news story on the radio as the nurse begins her day. She stops brushing her teeth to hear what the announcer is saying. She can't believe her ears. It's horrible.

The nurse reads about it while she eats breakfast. The story's on page three of the *Detroit Free Press*. There are pictures of you, Chris, and Jennifer. The nurse wonders how life can be so cruel.

In the halls of the hospital, the nurse talks with her co-workers. Isn't it terrible? If that poor Mr. Vandemark ever wakes up, how will he take the news? How sad.

✦✦✦✦

This news brought David back to consciousness. The nurse had noticed a solitary tear rolling down his cheek. Both cheeks were wet with tears by the time he was fully awake. The room was filled with doctors and nurses, all talking excitedly at him with both their minds and mouths. David Vandemark had regained consciousness, and everyone was on hand for the occasion. But their excited presences overwhelmed him, causing him to regress and forget everything he had learned about controlling his telepathy.

The voices thundered through his head, drowning out everything but the pain. Chris! Jenny! No! Oh, God! Stop! Stop everything! It was too unbearable. David Vandemark had performed the mental labors of Hercules in returning to the world, to find his entire life destroyed by a crazed knife-wielding butcher.

The excited babble continued unabated, but David was not strong enough to withstand its onslaught. One last look from inside a face ashen gray and streaked with tears, then he pulled the sheets over his head and began to sob. At this point his nurse took charge and abruptly hustled the others out of the room. The nurse dashed to the dispensary for a strong sedative, but David didn't notice their departure. He was rushing headlong toward oblivion. Gone. Everything he loved was gone. All that was left was the comforting void. He raced toward it, hoping it would put an end to pain and suffering. It did. David Vandemark died.

∞∞∞

David remembered his cigarette, which had burned down almost to his fingers, took a final drag, and stubbed it out in the little glass ashtray on the coffee table. Poor dead David Vandemark. For all his intelligence, David couldn't handle his strange new existence. That was why he had chosen death, had literally made himself die.

But Mother Nature, who abhors a vacuum, had spent a lot of time and effort putting David Vandemark back together. She had a good reason for doing this and would be damned if she'd see all her hard work go to waste. So when David decided to check out, she salvaged a piece of the emotional wreckage and nurtured it. Her plan was to have the fragment become the whole. She succeeded admirably. At least so it seemed at the time.

∞∞∞

Reawakening. A resurrection. Those were embarrassing memories. He hadn't handled the event well. It had been a time of transition, a changing of the guard. He wasn't certain when, during those chaotic two days, the new personality had emerged. He remembered only the tears, the gut-wrenching emotions, and hiding under the sheets. Were those David Vandemark's final torturous moments, or his birth traumas? Impossible to say.

The doctors were happy about his sudden recovery. They couldn't leave well enough alone, though. They wanted to regale him with details about what had happened. Their explanations were excruciatingly boring, since he already knew the nature of his injuries, but he humored his doctors. Dealing with them turned out to be more of a chore than he'd imagined. Few people can appreciate the mind-numbing effects of listening to people laboriously explain something when you've already gleaned the gist of it with a quick scan of their minds. It would take him time to get used to this. His new gift not only made conversation unnecessary but turned it into a burden, one he would have to shoulder if he wanted to remain among his fellow humans.

The hospital staff couldn't comprehend his desire to check out as soon as possible. He was afraid to remain, fearing they might discover the switch. Would Blue Cross cover his medical expenses if it was discovered that the insured had had an unauthorized personality transplant?

The new David Vandemark feared that a CAT scan or some other equally sophisticated medical examination might reveal a new set of brain waves. There would be no glib explanation of such a phenomenon. "Well it's like this, Doc. The old tenant didn't like the redecorating job you did on his head, so he split. I was passing by, just looking for a place to stay, and I loved what you'd done with it, so . . ."

The doctors would recommend only one prescription for this disorder: a one-way ticket to the booby hatch. David decided he could live without that, thanks.

The entire staff thought he was more than a little crazy and awfully rude when he insisted on leaving the hospital. They wanted to provide physical therapy, and they intended to run all sorts of tests. Once again David declined to go along with the program, but that didn't deter them. The doctors and nurses had one last trick up their sleeves.

It came as a terrible shock when their plans didn't meet with the expected results. Arthur Lowe's tearful revelation of the murder of Christine and Jennifer was old news to David. But the doctors didn't know this and couldn't figure out why David didn't fall to pieces. Well, why should he have? Sure, he shared all of David Vandemark's memories, but Chris and Jenny belonged to another life. Examining that past existence was like a voyeuristic experience to him. He was sorry they were dead in the same way that he'd feel bad, say, upon hearing of the death of a favorite television personality. The news did not touch him personally. The loss of Chris and Jenny had destroyed David Vandemark. His replacement would not let that happen.

Thinking of television reminded him of all the TV he'd watched while waiting to be released.

He knew he should have been thinking about his future. Going back to David Vandemark's dull existence was out of the question, but somehow the vast panorama of possibilities seemed too much to grasp all at once. With this newly discovered telepathic ability, decision-making had become more difficult. What couldn't he do now if he set his mind to it?

Better to chill in front of the tube for a while and marshal his energies before taking any drastic action. Tomorrow would be another day.

The afternoon glut of soap operas had driven him to watch Jimmy Swaggart on one of the local channels. At first he stayed with the show because he was amused by the preacher's bombast. Then, after the novelty wore off, he remained tuned in. Oddly enough, the words began to reach him.

When Swaggart went off the air, he found another religious program. The wonders of cable television. Over the next few days he caught every syndicated TV preacher the myriad stations had to offer. The nurses and doctors who came to his room saw this as a good sign. Poor David Vandemark, they thought, is gaining comfort from the words of the televised Bible. They had no idea how right they were.

Those Bible thumpers had shown him the light, all right. Oral Roberts, Jerry Falwell, Reverend Robert Schuller—they all spoke to him of the Lord, awakening within him something that David Vandemark had never suspected was there. It was an epiphany. A new beginning. Seeds falling on fertile soil and taking root. This newborn spiritualism grew within him like kudzu along a desolate southern road.

The preachers spoke of right and wrong. The political ideology they mixed with their religious messages stirred him. His path became clear. They had saved him long hours of soul-racking introspection. There would be no false starts, no doubts or worries. The television evangelists had shown him the way, opened his eyes to the truth. He had only one tiny reservation about these preachers: they tended to be a little too New Testament for his tastes. He had envisioned a more vengeful deity. God had to be vengeful. Why else would he, in his infinite wisdom, working hand in hand with Mother Nature, have created this new and improved David Vandemark?

And so David's replacement had been doing the Lord's work for the past seven years. It hadn't been an easy job, but it had certainly been rewarding.

David Vandemark took a small glass knickknack from a nearby bookshelf. Despite the fingerprint smudges, which showed that Angela had regularly handled this object, he picked up no reading. Not surprising, he thought. If he couldn't read Angela's mind, why should he expect to pick up impressions from something she'd touched? Not like those scissors. . . .

He had discovered his talent for reading residual psychic traces on objects while he was having a cast put on his leg at Beaumont Hospital. The technician had extracted a pair of scissors from his back pocket and set them on the table beside David. As he watched the man apply the cast, David had inadvertently brushed his hand against the scissors. The contact was like an electric shock.

It took him a few minutes to work up the courage to touch the scissors again. From this contact he learned that the technician was John Theakston, a Canadian who was working in this country illegally. He'd come to the States as a college student and decided to stay. His girlfriend was a waitress named Jill Nelson. He was cheating on her with one of her best friends.

The traces weren't nearly as clear and powerful as direct telepathic communication with a living subject. But these residual memories were much more detailed, perhaps because the subject's conscious mind was not interfering with his reading. The traces were neither obscured nor contained by a linear thought pattern.

David learned later on that this trick would work only with objects that had been in contact with a person over an extended time or during a period of high emotion. It took time for an inanimate object to pick up the essence of a person under normal circumstances. Psychometry— this ability to read inanimate objects—had come in very handy along the way. It was a very useful skill.

The man who replaced David Vandemark knew even before he left Beaumont Hospital that his psychic skills would lead him to Chris and Jenny Vandemark's killer. It was as if a sacred light now illuminated his path. It never occurred to him to inform the police that he could lead them to Mr. Clean. He knew the court system would merely imprison the killer and let him live out the rest of his days in the relative comfort of a cell with a color television. The media would create a ghoulish celebrity out of this monster. Clean would live to see his golden years, basking in his infamy, reveling in the fact that he was one of the new bogeymen.

No, that would never do.

And so one night, less than a week after his release from the hospital, David's replacement made his way clumsily but with unwavering determination to the basement of the Vandemark house. He did not turn on the lights. Some deeds were best left shrouded in darkness.

David could feel the smooth hardness of the tile floor beneath his feet. The basement smelled of mildew, laundry detergent, and kerosene. Dim light from the house next door filtered in through two small cellar windows. One shaft eerily lit the Magic Marker outline of a body. Chris's body. A chill ran through him, but it wasn't the dampness. David knew that no one, except perhaps another psychic, would be able to sense this effluvium. It was the essence of terror and death. He could smell it. Taste it. Feel it seeping into the pores of his skin. It nearly drove him out of the basement, but he overcame his revulsion, gritted his teeth, and limped toward the outline.

David had to sit uncomfortably on the floor to touch the place where the body had lain. He hesitated, his hand above the tiles, dreading what he was about to do. He closed his eyes, took a deep breath, and pressed his palm flat against the floor.

The contact hit him like a blow to the solar plexus. He raised his hand reflexively as a pathetic cry escaped his lips. One tiny touch had revealed volumes. The terrifying last moments of Chris Vandemark raced through his startled mind. Her pain, fear, humiliation, uncomprehending horror, sorrow, and death were now David's. He would share them with her for eternity. In the silent darkness of that basement, David swore to Chris that he would avenge her heinous murder.

The only thing he didn't know was the identity of the killer. He lowered his hand to the floor again, searching for another psychic trace, convinced that it was there and that he would recognize it. As he searched, other images of Chris surfaced; her life rolled before his unseeing eyes like a filmed documentary: her first kiss, her marriage to David, her high-school years, her dead mother and overly ambitious father, Jenny's birth. David felt tears in his eyes. But he felt something else as well. He was getting closer. It was more to the right. A presence. A chill. Farther forward. He kept searching.

Touching Chris's terror had been a jarring experience, a physical jolt. Contact with Mr. Clean, though, was another matter entirely. As soon as he touched the spot where Greg Hewett had knelt while sodomizing his victim, David felt himself falling, dropping into the black emotional void that was Mr. Clean. David shuddered violently as the blood drained from him. The evil was grafted onto his own soul during this, the first of many such encounters that David would have over the years as he hunted human monsters.

He'd had no idea of the depths of depravity a man could

sink to and still pass for normal. He'd never dreamed that such abominations walked among their fellow men. This was a totally unexpected horror. David had assumed that most people were like him, sharing a common morality that allowed the world to function without toppling into the abyss of chaos. He realized there was a wide range to that moral spectrum, that there were madmen who could no longer qualify as humans, but he was convinced that one could recognize them. Their insanity would make them stand out from the crowd. Their perceptions were so warped as to preclude anonymity.

What David felt now was beyond his comprehension. He was in touch with the psyche of a being that did not understand and was not bound by basic human mores. This creature made its way through life pretending to feel friendship, love, happiness, sorrow—the entire range of emotions. But there was a terrible nothingness where its soul should have been. Such an anomaly couldn't exist! God couldn't allow such a monster to walk the earth! It couldn't be true!

With a shuddering shriek, he pulled his hand away from the floor and sat there panting, his lungs burning, his eyes ablaze with the fire of new understanding. He had gazed into the flames of hell and seen the truth. The monster was real. The aberration walked the earth and David had never suspected its existence. Some part of David realized that Mr. Clean wasn't a unique creature. The beast had brethren.

❧❧❧

Back in Angela's apartment David marveled at what a quiet revolution this integration process had been. Yes, the king was dead. Long live the king. He was the old king we all thought had died. But he hadn't died, not really. He was only pretending to be the new king who just died. But he didn't die either. So I guess that means no one really died. We just thought they did. Luckily we were mistaken.

David knew he'd grasp it later. Trying to unravel it all now would only give him a headache.

What did matter was the way he felt, which was terrific! As if a great weight had been lifted. David would no longer have to fool himself into thinking that emotions never touched him. That indulgence had taken an incredible amount of energy. Energy he could put to better use.

No longer some unfeeling avenging angel, David Vandemark was once more an ordinary human being. He had a couple of clever tricks up his sleeve, but underneath the telepathic parlor games was David Vandemark, average citizen.

This realization, he decided, wouldn't change anything. He still had a job to do. God the Father, Mother Nature, or some other authoritative relative had given him this power and set him on the course he was currently navigating. He couldn't see any reason to change it. The work still needed to be done and he honestly couldn't think of anyone better suited for the job.

Maybe the old David Vandemark would not have been able to handle the incongruity of this situation—an average guy with an unorthodox, socially unacceptable talent—and would have promptly started looking for some covers to pull over his head. But this David Vandemark had seen the seamy underbelly of the human condition and had accepted it as simply another fact of life.

Listen, buddy, he reminded himself, someone's got to follow the circus parade and shovel the elephant shit. If you discover you've got a knack for it, why not? What are you going to do now, anyway? Go back to Bradhurst, Weiss, and Lowe?

Glancing toward Angela's bedroom, he contemplated the radical changes in attitude and persona that would have to accompany this new presence in his life. Maybe he had been going it alone for too long. It seemed the future had other things in store for him.

The man with many names and many personalities had jealously guarded his solitude, knowing that if he didn't get close to anyone, he wouldn't get hurt. But the midgame substitute had dropped the ball. Or perhaps he'd taken it as far as he could and needed a rest. A permanent vacation.

Whatever the reason, David had been pulled off the bench. It was time for him to call the shots again. He saw no reason to continue going it alone. Alone, David had spent seven years thinking he was at least two different people. Without someone at his side he might slip back into that delusion. He wasn't an island. He needed people, just as the old David Vandemark had needed . . .

The realization rolled over him with a fury he could not have anticipated. It left him gasping and feeling once more like a drowning man. He had been so busy thinking about the present that he had neglected to stave off the past, which even now was surging forward to catch up with him. He could not ward it off. It had been suppressed for too long.

So in the darkness of Angela Quinoñes's living room, David Vandemark wept for his wife and child, seven long years dead.

26

Angela had forgotten to set her alarm clock, so she and David didn't wake up until nine-thirty. In a hurried, half-awake call to her office she explained that she'd overslept but would be there within the hour.

David lay in bed next to her, smiling and feeling good. He enjoyed looking at her. Lord, she was beautiful. After hanging up the phone, Angela rolled back over to David. Their mouths found each other. The kiss was warm and filled with longing. David felt himself stir, but Angela reluctantly pulled away.

"Sorry, but we're putting the magazine to bed today. No way I can take the day off."

David gave her a peck on the forehead and playfully shoved her toward the edge of their warm burrow of sheets. "I understand completely. I've got a few things to do today myself. I'm on a manhunt. Remember?"

He could tell by the shadow that crossed Angela's lovely face, like a cloud passing over the sun, that she did. "Don't worry. I'm just going to check on that exterminator's van. Shouldn't be anything dangerous about that."

"Unless the driver turns out to be the Slasher," she said.

"I'm delighted that you're so concerned about my welfare, but the chances of that are pretty slim. Only TV cops find criminals so easy to track. If the van was somehow connected to the killings, it'll probably only lead me to a long series of other clues. My chances of meeting the Slasher today are practically nil."

Angela stared long and hard at David, trying to decide if he was telling the truth, but she couldn't read his deadpan expression. So she mentally shrugged her shoulders, gave him another quick kiss, and got out of bed.

David threw on a pair of pants and meandered out into the kitchen. By the time Angela had showered and dressed, he had breakfast waiting for her. Scrambled eggs, English muffins, juice, and coffee.

Angela was amazed. "Do you always treat your ladies this well?"

"Only when they're special. And then only when I'm starving."

There was some morning-after awkwardness at breakfast, both of them hoping not to say anything stupid, wanting to keep their cool and not give too much away. They had a hard time not looking too intently at each other, but they got past the bad moments with warm smiles and small talk. No talk of the Slasher. Or of love. It was too early even to think about such a thing, though the feeling was in the air.

David threw on the rest of his clothes and walked Angela to the subway station, where he kissed her good-bye and then watched her disappear among the successive waves of late-morning commuters.

David retraced his steps to the van, retrieved a small personal computer and a metal carrying case, closed up the vehicle, and returned to Angela's apartment.

On the way, he picked up the local newspapers. There was nothing new in them about the Slasher, but the *New York Times* carried a banner headline about the mayor being booed at a town meeting in Spanish Harlem. The protesters were incensed over the NYPD's lack of progress on the Slasher case. They contended that if the Slasher's victims had been white Anglo-Saxon Protestants, Jews, or African-Americans, the killer would have been brought to justice by now. Uninterested in hearing the mayor's excuses, they chanted "Justice for all, not just for whites!" until His Honor left the stage. David read the stories with a certain amount of amazement at the extent to which this case was polarizing the city.

❦❦❦❦

When he called the number on the side of the tan van, a computer informed him that the phone was no longer in service. There was no listing for Taglia Exterminators in the phone book or Yellow Pages, and Information was no help either. David wasn't exactly surprised.

He set up his computer. From the carrying case he produced a modem and connected it to the computer and a phone jack. He leafed through a notebook he kept in the case. This ring binder contained essential phone numbers, each of which was a treasured key. Collectively they enabled him to break into virtually any restricted database. David was very proud of his abilities as a hacker.

Before getting started, he hunted around the apartment until he found Angela's stationery. He addressed an envelope to Mrs. Rosita Vallejo. Into it he slipped twenty of the hundred-dollar bills he had won from Dominic Torres in Florida. He stuck a stamp on the envelope and dropped it in his sport coat pocket for mailing later. David smiled sardonically. Dominic wouldn't have cared a rat's ass about some poor woman who might end up living on the streets. There was tremendously satisfying irony in knowing his money was being used to prevent that from happening to Mrs. Vallejo.

Time to get to work. David's first move was to route his inquiries through cellular modems he had set up in backwoods shacks outside Minneapolis and Denver. This would make it impossible for most computer security experts to track down the perpetrator of the criminal trespass David was about to commit. Sure, a security supersleuth like Tsutomu Shimomura could eventually track David down, but for the files Vandemark planned to rifle through, nobody would bother to hire an expert.

Looking into the central Public Assistance database allowed David to confirm his suspicion that all of the Slasher's victims had, in fact, been on welfare at one time. Not exactly the breakthrough he was looking for, but at least it was another piece of the puzzle. And David knew that when there were enough pieces, the picture would at last make sense.

The phone company database had no listing for Taglia Exterminators, so David decided to look for a registration on the van. But the odds were good that if the Slasher used the vehicle on his bloody forays, he wouldn't risk being stopped by the police.

How would it look if a cop pulled over a van that said Taglia Exterminators on the side but was registered to a Sam Smith? Maybe our boy would explain it away deftly, but the cop would remember, especially if there had been a murder that night anywhere in the vicinity. The Slasher couldn't chance that. Everything so far indicated that this psycho was a good planner. Damn good. He'd cover himself somehow.

The DMV's computer came up empty on Taglia, so he searched for the van itself.

It took some doing to get the system to kick out a list of all the tan vans registered in the state. David was horrified at the number of similar vehicles that were running around. Why was it he didn't see one or two of them on every block?

Again, no Taglia Exterminators or Taglia anything else among the multitude of names. The van could be registered to a holding company with another name. But that would leave the Slasher with the same set of problems he'd have had with a vehicle registered to Sam Smith: the name and the vehicle would be remembered.

David remembered that Angela had described the van as light brown at first, as if she'd had trouble translating Mrs. Vallejo's description. On a hunch, David punched in "brown."

Under the S listings he found Sal Taglia Enterprises. The registration showed a 1985 Chevy van. A cop would have had to be Sherlock Holmes to notice the color distinction. It would look like a clerical error. Later on, if asked to check tickets issued on the night of the murder, the officer would likely say "No tan vans. Had one brown van, but no tans."

Sal Taglia Enterprises had a West Side address. That's odd, thought David. Nothing that far west except derelict warehouses and docks. Another dead end?

At first Taglia Enterprises didn't look promising. David parked across from the riverfront warehouse and glumly surveyed its boarded-up shabbiness. It looked abandoned. He turned off the ignition, got out, opened the van's hood, and began pretending to be a stranded motorist. While fiddling under the hood, David studied the turn-of-the-century white elephant across the street.

As he slammed the hood closed, a cab pulled up in front of the warehouse. A man in a navy suit got out and entered the building. The cab glided away from the curb and kept going. David got back in his vehicle and drove away. Experience told him something was very wrong here.

What kind of business chose to set up shop in a crummy neighborhood like this and didn't put up a sign to let the public know where it was? Why wasn't the company listed in the phone book? And what exactly did Sal Taglia Enterprises do? Lots of questions and no answers. David decided a man in a parked van wasn't going to unlock the secrets of Sal Taglia Enterprises. But someone less conspicuous might.

27

Chester Pinyon knew he had one of the most boring jobs on the face of the earth, but he didn't care. The money was good and the hours afforded him time to pursue his true calling: painting. Chester's dream was to become a high-priced SoHo artist, get rich, and retire to a fabulous estate on Long Island Sound where he would enjoy a parade of adoring wives and mistresses and live to a ripe old age creating masterpieces just like Picasso. Chester wasn't planning to follow that master's stylistic footsteps. Au contraire. He was going to concentrate all his energies on pure abstraction. That was where the big bucks were. Look at how much a Jackson Pollock went for these days. Those abstract expressionists knew what they were doing. Of course Pollock had the slight advantage of being dead, but Chester was quite convinced he could achieve the same acclaim while living. After all, fame was his destiny.

In the meantime he paid his dues, not to mention his rent, by sitting in front of this godforsaken bank of closed-circuit television screens. Twenty glowing units stared back at him as he sat at his console. The work was mind-numbing, but Chester had learned during his eighteen months on the job that if he scanned all the screens at once he could achieve a restful alpha state in which he was conscious but almost in a trance. Very Zen. He'd leave his shift thoroughly relaxed, his creative juices flowing. His meditation didn't interfere at all with his efficiency on the job. If anything unusual appeared on any of the monitors, some part of his subconscious would rouse him. He'd note it in the logbook or call Mr. Camden if it smelled like trouble.

This was the perfect job for an undiscovered genius, even though he couldn't understand why this warehouse had such an elaborate security system. Jesus, the place was a dump. Who'd want to rob it? Of course, the main offices might be really nice, Chester supposed, but his security clearance allowed him access only to the ground-floor security offices and the coffee room next door.

He knew this facility was connected with the government, but his knowledge and his curiosity both ended there. When Chester was hired, Mr. Camden had assured him that he'd be happy during his stay with their organization as long as he obeyed a few simple regulations. The most important of these was that he never ask questions or speak of his work to anyone on the outside. That suited Chester fine. Scuttlebutt had it that the place was some sort of Middle East think tank. That was all right with him too. He wasn't political. As long as they kept paying him the big bucks, these guys could do whatever they wanted and he would never breathe a word about it.

The reason he'd never dream of breaking Charles Camden's prime directive was Camden himself, a man who scared the shit out of Chester. The man had never been anything but polite and civil to him, but that didn't keep Chester from feeling a chill every time he saw his boss. There was something about the man that flashed an invisible warning. No bluster or bullying were needed to convey this. The threat was much more subtle than that.

Mr. Camden had left the security room a short while ago, so Chester was a little on edge. That was why he didn't notice the beat-up black van on monitor number seven right away. Its driver was poking around in the engine compartment. At least it gave Chester something to watch for a while. Maybe a tow truck would be called. That would be nice.

As Chester savored the prospect of a shift enlivened by some free entertainment, he punched commands into the console's computerized video center. The camera on number seven zoomed in on the vehicle. Chester jotted down the truck's license number in the logbook. Standard practice. He panned with the camera to get a look at the van's owner. The guy looked like a Latino. It figured. Those types drove around in either gaudy Caddies or junkers. It had probably been years since that clunker had passed a safety inspection without the examiner being slipped a few bucks.

Chester was surprised and disappointed when the man jumped back into his truck and drove off. He logged the van's departure time, then settled into his usual trancelike state. Nothing new disturbed him until Jerry Stillson tapped him on the shoulder a half hour later and told him to go to lunch. Jerry, his relief today, asked if anything was happening. "Does anything ever happen on this job?" Chester replied. "Why should today be any different?"

28

David Vandemark parked his van in a public garage five blocks from the warehouse. He wanted it off the street. The warehouse had spooked him. There was something fishy about the joint. David wanted his wheels out of sight but handy in case he had to make a run for it.

He changed into some ragged clothes he'd brought along for such an eventuality. New York's streets were filled with homeless people. One more could join their ranks without being noticed. The only difference was that this one would be packing a 9 mm Smith & Wesson under his tattered raincoat.

As David walked out of the garage, the parking attendant stared at him, confused. The man who'd arrived in the van a few minutes ago hadn't been dressed like that. David flashed his parking stub.

A half block from the garage David spotted a puddle near the curb. It was perfect—full of mud, crud, and city grime, topped off with an oily rainbow. He dipped his hands into the mess and rubbed the slime into his scalp and onto his neck and face as passersby looked on in horrified fascination. They'd have a great story to tell at the office after lunch.

Ten minutes later, his disguise dried and rubbed to a fine patina, David returned to the warehouse. He approached the south end, from behind a neighboring derelict structure. That building was definitely abandoned. Its windows had been knocked out, and it was a real hell hole inside. David wandered seemingly without direction. Poking into doorways, examining the ground for oracles or spare change. He made a point of giving the object of his interest merely an occasional passing glance while keeping it under observation the rest of the time in his peripheral vision. There was no telling at this distance if someone might be watching him.

He shambled over to a Dumpster and saw that it was empty; there'd been a pickup this morning.

He went around to the front of the building but found no clue to what went on in there. If someone had come out he could have gotten a reading off them, but no such luck.

The north side of the warehouse revealed only an empty parking lot closed off with a chain. From there David could see that the warehouse hung out over the water, supported by cement stanchions and timber pilings. There didn't appear to be any activity here, either.

Feeling more brazen, David openly inspected the warehouse as he continued his tour of the exterior. He crossed to the far side of the street when he reached the front. This time he concentrated on the second floor and roof of the structure. The windows on that level had been boarded shut. That should have tipped him off from the beginning. None of the other buildings along this waterfront skid row had been boarded up tight to keep out prying eyes. It was a good camouflage job.

A glint of light bounced off something on the roof. David stopped dead in his tracks. He noticed the devices planted at regular intervals along the rooftop. Camouflaged to blend in with their deteriorating surroundings, some were tucked behind phony vent pipes, others hidden under loose shingles and other debris.

Now what? As David took a few paces south, hoping to get a better view of those strange contraptions, he noticed a box on a nearby lamppost. A round object made of glass was sticking out of one end. A video camera, probably, and it was pointed east, down the side street.

Those were cameras on the roof too. Smile! You're on Candid Camera.

Aw, Christ.

❧

Jerry Stillson had followed David's progress around the perimeter of the installation and simply noted his presence in the logbook. A bum passing through the area was nothing new. It happened at least once or twice a week. When they discovered pickings were slim, they usually moved on.

But this one didn't. He circled to the far north side of the building and then circled back to the south again. Worse yet, the bum seemed to be looking directly at the building as he completed his circuit. Jerry dialed Mr. Camden's line and waited for an answer.

Charles Camden picked up on the third ring. All he said was "Yes?"

Jerry replied as calmly as he could: "It appears we have someone interested in the installation, sir."

"I'll be right there."

Camden walked into the security office less than sixty seconds later. "What have you got?"

Stillson explained the situation, and the two men watched the twin screens that showed the trespasser staring intently at the building.

"Looks like he's wondering if he can get in here. Probably looking for a dry place to spend the night," said Camden.

With an ingratiating smile, Jerry Stillson replied, "He's picked the wrong place this time, hasn't he, sir?"

Charles Camden pressed a button on the control console and said more to himself than to Stillson, "Most definitely."

Ten seconds later two men in ill-fitting sport coats stepped into the security office. Both were large and burly, with thick necks and very little intelligence in their eyes.

Camden pointed to the two screens showing the intruder. "We've got an uninvited guest out front. I believe he's thinking about moving in. Gentlemen, dissuade him of that notion."

Pete Braddock and his partner, Joe Bates, smiled, then turned and left the room with such enthusiasm they almost knocked over Chester Pinyon, who was returning from lunch. When Chester noticed Mr. Camden in the room he felt his blood pressure jump twenty points. "Anything going on?" he asked timidly.

Jerry answered over his shoulder, "Evicting a tramp before he asserts squatter's rights."

Chester breathed a sigh of relief. False alarm. For a second there he'd thought he might have screwed up something on his shift and that all the commotion was about rectifying it, but this sort of thing had happened before. Count to ten and shut down the adrenaline factory. He sat down next to Jerry, picked up the log, and read about what he had missed during lunch.

Watching the dual screens overhead, Charles Camden and Jerry saw Braddock and Bates approach the bum, who was now sitting on the curb as if he didn't have a care in the world. Camden grinned. That fool tramp had no idea the entire world was about to come crashing in on him.

Braddock grabbed the bum by his collar and hauled him to his feet. As the vagrant rose, Bates laid a fist into his stomach. Braddock then slammed the tramp into the front of the building across the street. The two guards tossed the derelict back and forth for a moment, then Braddock punched him in the eye and he went down like a sack of potatoes. Bates grabbed the bum by the ear and convinced him to stand, while Braddock delivered the coup de grâce, a good kick to the backside, which sent him on his way. Camden could well imagine the threats his boys were imparting. If they ever found him in this neighborhood again, he wouldn't get off so easy.

"*Holy Shit!* That's the guy from this morning!"

Camden spun to face Chester, who was pointing at the twin monitors.

"What are you talking about, Pinyon?"

"That man was hanging around here earlier! He was in a van!"

"Are you sure it's the same person?"

"Positive! He was dressed differently, but that's the same guy!"

Camden was furious. Braddock and Bates didn't carry hand radios. There was no way to countermand his previous orders. So his hired goons were standing in the middle of the street, blithely watching the bum stumble off. In a calm, matter-of-fact voice Camden said, "Stillson, run outside and tell Bates and Braddock that I want that man brought to my office immediately."

Stillson tore off like a champion sprinter, but Camden knew he would be too late. The trespasser was already rounding the corner. Camden shifted his gaze to another monitor. As he had suspected, as soon as the derelict was out of view of Braddock and Bates, he straightened up and began to run like an Olympic hopeful. He'd be down the block and out of sight before Stillson ever reached the street. There was probably a car waiting for the spy. Further pursuit would be useless.

Camden instructed Pinyon to log the incident and then left the security office. Who did the spy work for? Local police? FBI? CIA? Maybe one of the newspapers? How had they tumbled to his setup? And more important, how much did they know? Not much, judging from the fact that they were only beginning to nose around the outside of the installation. But now that they had the scent there'd be no shaking them.

That meant the timetable would have to be moved up. He had hoped for at least three more test runs. Now they would have to satisfy themselves with one final rehearsal. This was regrettable, of course, but not critical. The desired results of this exercise had been achieved. New York's Hispanic community was in an uproar over the killings. Camden had seen the look of fear in the eyes of Latinos he'd passed on the street. Their leaders were harassing City Hall, demanding that something be done about the murders. Hispanic faith in the city government was eroding daily. They were calling for outside investigators. Anarchy had not yet seized control of the city, but it was brewing nicely.

Camden reached into his shirt pocket for a cigarette as he watched Braddock and Bates enter the room. Both looked nervous and ashamed. Braddock fished around in his clothes for his lighter; someone had told him that was how one curried favor with one's superiors. Camden enjoyed the man's toadying.

"I'm sorry, Chief. By the time we got word, the creep was gone," Bates said as he and his partner stepped out of Camden's way. Braddock was still hunting around for his lighter.

Camden pulled out his own and lit the cigarette. Pete Braddock looked crestfallen, as if missing this light on top of losing the bum added up to kissing his next promotion good-bye. Or worse. "Can't seem to find my lighter. Had it a while ago."

"Ya probably dropped it when we was waltzing around with the spick," Bates offered.

"Yeah, let's go check. That was a Zippo, cost me ten bucks."

As the two men turned to go, Camden noticed that Bates was missing a button on his sport jacket.

᧥᧥᧥

David Vandemark tossed the lighter and the button into a trash can. The two objects had told him all they could. His attackers had been Joe Bates and Pete Braddock, both ex-pugs, now working as security guards at Sal Taglia Enterprises. Neither knew what kind of work Sal Taglia Enterprises did, but both suspected it had something to do with the government. Most of the time all they did was sit in the waiting room, playing cards and watching television. Every other week or so they'd be called on to roust some bum.

David had gleaned from the items a lot of other useless information about the hired thugs' business and private lives. But only one fact held any interest for him: the name of their supervisor was Charles Camden.

29

Angela returned from work that evening tired from her day's labors but energized by the thought that Leroy might be there when she got home. She had promised herself she wouldn't be disappointed if he wasn't. After all, he was in town on a job. There was no telling what his hours might be.

Besides, what would she say to him if he was there? How should she act toward him? Last night had been sheer ecstasy, and she knew it had been as good for him. But it didn't mean much. Neither of them had made any vows of undying love. They had simply spent a night together. Consenting adults did that all the time without moving on to wedded bliss.

Wedded bliss? Angela hardly knew the guy! He could be a slob and a drunk for all she knew. Leroy might like to beat his women once he had them broken in. He could even be a pimp, maybe looking for a new recruit.

Angela smiled at that notion. The thought of Leroy driving around in a big pink Cadillac was a deliciously ludicrous image. There was an overwhelming gentleness about the man.

As she reached the door of her apartment, she heard movement within. Her heart skipped a beat. She took a deep breath, unlocked the door, and stepped in. But the first thing she saw were his sport coat and shoulder holster resting on one of the living-room chairs. So what kind of gentleman carried a gun?

That thought vanished when she heard a voice call from the kitchen: "Angela? I'm in here."

He was sitting at the kitchen table, his back to her. On the table was a personal computer; her phone was connected to it.

"Where did that come from?" she asked.

"From my van. I'm afraid I'm running up your phone bill."

"That's okay. But what are you . . . *Jesus Christ!*"

David had turned around as she was speaking. His right eye was slightly swollen and in the process of turning a lovely shade of purple. Angela felt her heart drop into her shoes. "What happened? Are you all right?"

David stood up and gave her a hug. "I'm fine. Just a little bruised."

"What happened?"

"Got a bit careless. Let myself get maneuvered into a bad situation, and two gorillas worked me over a bit. I could have stopped them, but it wouldn't have looked right. So I rolled with a few punches and got what might prove to be some very useful information."

Angela gently touched David's swollen brow. "I can see you did a great job of rolling with those punches."

"Well, that one came out of left field. Wasn't prepared for it."

Heading for the refrigerator, Angela said, "You need some ice on that eye."

"Good idea. I should have thought of that myself, but I've been kind of busy."

As she wrapped a washcloth around some ice, Angela asked, "What are you doing on that thing?" She nodded toward the computer.

"That *thing*? Don't you use a computer at work?"

"As little as possible. I don't trust those machines. I never know when our system's going to crash. Fortunately my new assistant practically lives on the Internet."

"Well, the times they are a-changing, my dear woman, so don't be too surprised if one day your relationship with the computer changes as well."

"That may be. In the meantime, why don't you tell me about your current affair with this particular machine."

David pressed the ice pack to his brow. "I'm trying to learn something about a man, but I'm not getting very far."

"Who's the man? Someone involved in this case?"

A thin, reedy silence fell, during which Angela could feel the barriers sliding into place. After an interminable pause David said a bit awkwardly, "This job is turning into more than I bargained for."

"What do you mean?"

"When I've had cases like this in the past they've been pretty straightforward. All I had to do was hunt down the bad guy and bag him. It's not working out that way this time around. Some very strange players are popping up in the game."

Angela thought that over. "What are you trying to tell me?"

"I'm trying to say that things are getting complicated. I'm not sure where this case is heading. This is a new experience for me. Usually with this type of job I've got everything pretty much under control. But not this time. That worries me."

"Are you in any kind of trouble, Leroy?"

"Not yet. At least I don't think so. I handled today's little fiasco without getting anyone on my tail. But I might not be so lucky next time, so I've decided to take some precautions."

David picked up a sealed envelope from the kitchen table and handed it to Angela. She could feel an odd rectangular shape inside it. The envelope was addressed to an Ira Levitt in care of the FBI. "What's this?"

"An audiocassette. On it I've recorded everything I've learned about this case so far. I don't want to be melodramatic and I don't want to scare you, but I want some backup in case anything happens to me. I don't know anyone else in this town I can trust, so I'm afraid you've been elected."

Angela looked at the bulging envelope in her hand. "In other words, if you don't show up here some night I'm to mail this off?"

"Exactly."

"What's on this tape?"

"It's best you don't know. If anything blows up in my face, someone from the government might track my movements to you. If you don't know anything other than the fact that you mailed a tape for me, they won't hassle you."

"Jesus, Leroy! The government! What are you into?"

David patted her hand gently. "I wish I knew, and I

wish I could tell you. But I can't. That's the way it's got to be."

He watched Angela walk woodenly from the kitchen. After a few moments he followed. He found her curled up on the sofa in the living room, looking out the window unhappily. David stood there scrutinizing her.

How could he have been so stupid as to get her involved in this? The man with a thousand names had been right. There was no place in this life for a woman. It was too dangerous. "Maybe it would be best if I went and found that hotel room."

"No. That wouldn't help. I'd go out of my mind worrying about you. At least this way I'll know you're all right while you're here. I'm sorry, Leroy, but you've become part of my life. I care about you. I don't want to see anything happen to you."

David sat down and put an arm around her. "I care for you too, a lot more than I would have thought possible in such a short time."

This elicited a faint smile from Angela. She leaned closer and quickly kissed him. The kiss didn't last long, but David could sense the urgency in it before she buried her face in his shoulder. Though he couldn't see them, he knew the tears were there. They scalded his heart.

In a weak voice Angela said, "If you can't find the information on this man you're hunting . . . what will you do? Can you at least tell me that?"

"I guess so. He's got some connection with the government. That much I know. Must be in some organization with direct links to the upper echelons of power. I accessed local FBI computer records, but I was informed that his file was sealed. Had no idea how to break into it without having the line traced back to your phone. The Feds are kind of touchy about unauthorized entry."

"Does that mean you've hit a dead end?" Angela asked, something like hope in her voice.

"No, it means I've got to go through a back door. In this case that back door happens to be an FBI agent named Johnson."

"Is this agent a friend of yours?"

"Not exactly. We're business acquaintances. I'm having lunch with her tomorrow, as a matter of fact."

"What are you doing tonight?"

"Absolutely nothing. Thought I'd sit around here with my favorite lady and see if the ice pack will take down the swelling on my eye. How's that sound?"

"*Bueno.* Why don't we go into the bedroom, Leroy."

"Sounds like a great idea. But first, would you do me a favor?"

"What's that?"

"Don't call me Leroy. I use my middle name professionally. I'd rather you used my first name."

"Which is?"

"David."

30

Charles Camden sat back in his chair, exhausted. His normally bare desk was a jumble of half-eaten take-out food, hastily scrawled notes, and open Rolodex files. He'd been working the phone all afternoon, talking to contacts at different federal and state agencies, trying to find out who was sniffing around his West Side operation. The existence of his outfit was an open secret among Washington's power elite, but its exact purpose was known only to a select few. If he could find out which agency was snooping, he could warn them off.

He wasn't worried that his inquiries would start people wondering what he was up to in New York. All of the contacts he talked to were deep in Camden's debt and would be circumspect in their investigations. He had instructed them to call back the minute they learned anything. That meant spending the next twenty-four hours or so by the phone. Sleeping on the office sofa. It was a small price to pay if it put a lid on this mess.

The license number on the black mystery van had been of no use to him. The Illinois DMV informed him that no such number had ever been issued in their state. Camden wasn't surprised.

He had given that tag number to long-time associates of his on the NYPD whom he trusted to handle the matter discreetly. He wanted them to find the van and inform him of its location; they were to take no action against the vehicle or its owner. This was an internal security matter that Camden's people could handle.

That was another call that might come at any time.

The intercom lit up, and Camden pressed a button on the speaker phone. "Yes?"

"McGuire and Hanson to see you, Mr. Camden."

"Send them in."

A moment later McGuire and Hanson stepped into the office. Camden enjoyed watching these men enter a room. No matter how many times they'd been here, they always came through the door alert and ready for trouble. Every doorway might be a trap as far as these two were concerned. Camden had taught them to respond that way. He'd taught them well.

He gestured to the two chairs in front of his desk. Hanson and McGuire took that as an invitation to be seated. Each man carried a manila envelope. Camden extended a hand. "Those are your reports on Alfredo Martinez and Esteban Moreno? Are they complete?"

Both men nodded and handed over the envelopes. He placed them in a desk drawer without looking at them. "Have you gentlemen any plans for this evening?"

The two men shook their heads.

"I may need your services on a rush job. I'd appreciate it if you'd stay on call throughout the night. Find yourselves a couple bunks down in the dorm, okay?"

Both men nodded, then got up and left the office.

Good men.

Camden spent the next hour going over reports that needed his attention. The phone rang twice. Both calls were from Washington contacts reporting they'd found nothing. Camden thanked them, hung up, and returned to his paperwork.

The third call was from one of Camden's friends at the NYPD. The black Ford Econoline he was looking for had been spotted in a public garage on Twenty-seventh Street. Two officers in a patrol car were keeping an eye on it. Camden instructed the sergeant to call off the patrol. His people would take over surveillance duties immediately. Camden assured his friend that there would be a packet hand-delivered to him tomorrow and hung up.

He got on the intercom and called the installation's barracks. When the attendant answered, Camden said, "Ask Mr. McGuire and Mr. Hanson to join me in my office. Tell them their job came through."

31

At 8:20 A.M. Vida glanced up from the Latino Family Killer file and reached for her lukewarm, bitter coffee, her third cup. Noticing Ira's dark expression, she followed his gaze out the door of the file room at One Police Plaza and saw a burly man in an ill-fitting sport coat, handing the desk sergeant a manila envelope. "Something wrong, Ira?"

"Probably," mumbled Ira. "But it's none of our business."

"The gorilla in the awful sport coat?"

Ira nodded almost imperceptibly. "Goon named Bates. Freelance muscle, hires out mostly within the spook community. The guy Bates usually works for is a particularly nasty piece of work."

"Any connection to our case?"

"Different world entirely," Ira said, returning to his file. "I'm more worried about this lawyer who called you. Run it through for me again."

Vida didn't mask her exasperation. This was the fourth time Ira had asked her to repeat the story. "He called my hotel room about six-forty-five last night. He said he had some information that might relate to our investigation.

Would I meet him for lunch? I tried to press him for some details, but he claimed he had to run. He hung up as I was about to ask him how he knew what we were investigating. That's the whole story, Ira, and it's the last time I'm going to tell it."

Ira was absentmindedly trying to scratch under his cast with a pencil. "I don't like it. First you tell me this Colson's trying to cozy up. Then all of a sudden he's got a lead for us. How'd he know which hotel we were staying at, anyway?"

"Lieutenant Nyberg probably told him. Remember, we informed Nyberg where we could be reached."

"Okay, okay,!" Ira conceded. "But what does Colson know about our case? What could he have found out about Vandemark that all our footwork hasn't uncovered?"

"Is that what's eating you, Ira? You're bent out of shape because our investigation turned up zip and you can't stand the thought of someone handing us a lead on a silver platter?"

Ira's face was a caricature: sullen lower lip out so far it was almost resting on the table. He stared at her, exuding displeasure, as Vida felt herself flush. Oops! she thought. Looks like I hit the nail on the head with that one. Not very diplomatic of me.

Finally Ira shook his head and said, "Maybe that's part of it. I don't know. But something about this doesn't feel right. Think I'll join you and Colson for that lunch."

32

This time Angela had remembered to set the alarm, so there was nothing hurried about her third morning with David. They took their time getting ready and lingered over breakfast, which Angela insisted on preparing. She claimed that the eggs David had made the previous day were overdone. Feigning hurt feelings, David kept Angela company, teasing her as she slaved over a hot stove.

When he kissed her good-bye at the Twenty-eighth Street subway entrance, David could see the worry in Angela's eyes. He wished he could dispel it, but he knew that anything he might do, short of quitting the case, would only be a stopgap measure. Better to get this Slasher mess behind them and let their future together unfold from there. Any thought that the man with a thousand names might have been right about going it alone had faded without a trace during last night's lovemaking.

Angela visibly willed a smile onto her face, tweaked his cheek, and disappeared rapidly down the subway steps.

David returned to his van, which was now parked in a public garage on Twenty-seventh Street. He had decided it would be wise to cover his tracks, and his first step had been to get his wheels out of sight as best he could. He'd informed the attendant on duty that he'd be coming back regularly to get things out of the van. The attendant had said there'd be no trouble as long as David always produced his stub when he came by. The van was on the roof level of the garage.

Inside the van, away from prying eyes, David changed into Jason Colson's gray three-piece suit, checked the lawyer's ID, and pocketed a twin-barreled .38 caliber derringer. Things had gotten too strange for Jason Colson, Justice Department lawyer, to walk around without firepower.

David armed the alarm, locked the van, and headed for the street. As he stopped to adjust his collar and cuffs, he had no inkling that Nelson McGuire was watching him from a nearby rooftop through a pair of high-magnification binoculars. McGuire signaled his partner on a hand radio that their quarry was on the move. Bud Hanson was already beating feet downstairs two at a time to pick up the tail at street level.

David headed toward the nearest subway station. His watch said 9:20; he had some two hours to run some important errands before his lunch date with Ira and Vida.

Half a block behind David, Bud Hanson was busy being invisible. A pro, he left plenty of space between himself and the pigeon. Hanson didn't know it, of course, but this was more than enough distance to keep him out of David's telepathic range.

Unaware of the bird dog on his trail, David trotted down into the subway station, graceful and dapper as Fred Astaire. He fished a token out of his pocket and slipped through the turnstile without any waiting. If he had looked over his shoulder, he might have noticed one of his fellow commuters rushing down the steps. But it would have meant nothing to him, triggered no alarms. What was one more harried New Yorker late for work? There was nothing striking about the man. Nothing sinister. Nothing worth remembering, in fact. That was what made Bud Hanson so ideal for the work he did.

A train was about to pull out as he stepped onto the platform. Three quick steps brought David into a car, the doors closed behind him, and the train pulled out without delay.

That was how David Vandemark lost his shadows without ever knowing they were there. Bud Hanson stood on the platform, watching the train disappear into the tunnel. No problem. They'd pick up this character again when he returned to his van.

33

Ira and Vida arrived half an hour early for their eleven-thirty lunch appointment. The waiter seated them at a quiet table near the back. The establishment's only other patrons at this hour were a couple of businessmen deep in fiscal discussion. Vida ordered a club soda to sip on while she waited for Colson. Ira would order later. As soon as the waiter departed, Ira headed toward the rest rooms.

He spotted a pair of pay phones outside the lavatories. This vantage point afforded him a clear view of Vida at the table. Satisfied with the layout, Ira lumbered into the men's room.

A scowl played across Ira's features as he relieved himself at a urinal. Ever since he'd heard about this lunch invitation from Colson, Ira's kishkes had been screaming that this was a setup. They hadn't settled down in the least after Ira had made a couple of calls to contacts in Washington. Turned out there was no Jason Colson in Justice. There was a John Colson, but he was currently assigned to a labor-racketeering task force in Chicago. Someone was using a false identity.

As if that wasn't bad enough, this someone was stepping on Ira's turf.

After washing his hands, Ira made sure he was alone in the rest room. He pulled out his piece, checked its load for the third time, and returned it to its holster.

Vida caught Ira's eye as he returned to the hallway. Her drink had arrived and, as previously arranged, Vida would remain at the table, sipping it. As far as anyone else was concerned, this lovely lady was simply waiting for her lunch date to arrive. Only Ira knew that her 9 mm automatic was resting in her lap, concealed by the tablecloth.

Ira picked up the handset of one of the pay phones and wedged it firmly between his ear and shoulder. He rummaged through his pockets. Where the hell were those Tums? A phone rang somewhere near the front of the restaurant as Ira located the Tums and cracked open the roll.

Before he could get one of the tablets to his mouth, Vida's waiter had stepped up to the table and handed her a box wrapped in plain brown paper. Ira slammed the receiver down on the cradle and stormed over. "What the hell's this!" he demanded.

Taken aback by the angry giant who'd raced up to him, the waiter stammered, "Just—just a package, sir. It was dropped off earlier."

"By whom?" asked Ira as he picked up the offending object.

"A gentleman came in as we were opening. He asked if he could leave it here for a friend who'd be stopping in for lunch. Said it was a birthday present."

"What did he look like?"

The waiter described David Vandemark. Ira looked to Vida for confirmation.

"Except for the swollen eye, that sounds like Colson," she said.

"Did he describe this friend of his?"

"No, I didn't even know his friend was a woman. The man said his friend would ask for the package."

"I didn't ask for anything," said Vida.

"No, you didn't." The waiter was totally flustered by now. "The gentleman called on the house phone and asked me to give the package to you."

"Did he ask if I was here first?" asked Vida.

"No."

Vida and Ira exchanged glances, then turned to the picture window fronting the street. "You've been very helpful," said Ira. The waiter relaxed visibly. "Can you bring me a glass of water?"

The waiter hurried off, leaving the package on the table.

"Should we call in the bomb squad?" Vida asked.

Ira looked up. "No, you can open it while I go to the john and lock myself in a stall."

"You don't have to get surly about—"

"Jesus!" Ira nearly fell over the table behind him, and Vida dropped her gun on the floor in her rush to get away from the table.

The mystery package was ringing.

"You're not going to open it, are you?" gasped Vida as Ira lunged forward and grabbed the package.

"Bombs don't ring, at least not like that. There's a phone in there. Someone's gotten shy on us."

Ira had the attention of everyone in the restaurant.

The businessmen had ceased their solemn discussion to see what the commotion was all about. The waiter, returning with Ira's water, stopped short and watched his large, surly customer rip open the mysterious package. No one saw Vida retrieve her gun from the floor.

There were two cellular phones inside the box, carefully padded with crumpled newspaper. They continued their persistent ringing. Ira pulled one out, examined it, and handed it to Vida. He picked up the other and answered it. "Hello, Mr. Colson. Where are you?"

"Hi, Ira," David answered via the wonder of modern technology. "How's the arm?"

"Itches all the time." Ira had never heard this voice before, but he knew exactly whom it belonged to. "And it still hurts like hell, you putz." Cupping the phone's mouthpiece, Ira whispered, "Get on the line. It's Vandemark."

As soon as Vida flipped on her phone she was greeted by "Sorry about standing you up, Vida. But I'm sure you understand."

"What's going down, Vandemark?" asked Ira. "This your way of turning yourself in?"

"Don't be absurd, Ira. Why would I do that?"

Rising to his feet, Ira walked to the front of the restaurant and scanned the street through the plate-glass window. "It's been seven years, David. It can't have been easy on you." There were two pay phones on the nearest corner. Neither was in use. At the far corner, down the street, a bank of three more phones. Two of them busy. At the first one, a lady with her back to Ira. Beyond her, someone else—someone Ira couldn't see because the woman was in the way.

Had to be Vandemark. He had to have seen them enter the restaurant.

"Think I'm getting tired, Ira?"

"Maybe."

"Well, you're right. But you can forget about my giving up."

Ira turned and signaled Vida. She understood and, without missing a beat, said into the phone, "From what I've read of your file, Mr. Vandemark, you're not one to play silly games. What are you up to?"

Covering the mouthpiece with his beefy hand, Ira whispered to the waiter, "Is there a rear exit? And where does it lead?" The waiter, sensing Ira's urgency and being terribly aware of Ira's monumental size, was thinking on his feet. "Yes. Out onto the alley. To Forty-third Street."

"I have a favor to ask of you," Vandemark said.

"The only favor you'll get from me, Vandemark, is a first-rate shrink once we have you behind bars," Ira barked.

"You might change your mind about that when you hear me out."

Ira signaled Vida once more before disappearing into the restaurant's kitchen. Over the phone she heard Ira say, "Screw you, Vandemark. The only thing I'm interested in is—"

"That's enough, Ira. Let me handle this," Vida said. "David, speak your piece."

A pause, then Vandemark said, "That's more like it. Let's talk straight for a couple of minutes, shall we?"

Out in the alley behind the restaurant, Ira growled into the phone, "Talk straight with you? You're a killer, Vandemark!"

"Ira, let the man talk!" commanded Vida in the toughest tone she could muster as she eyed the street; Ira had to be heading toward those three pay phones. "Let's hear what he has to say."

"Good idea, Vida. In fact, how about letting me do most of the talking. All you two have to do is grunt occasionally to let me know you're paying attention. Think you can handle that?"

A clear, high "Okay" and a deep-throated grunt were his answers. Ira proceeded down the alley.

"We've all been around long enough to know that some things in this world are more important than others," David said. "You with me?"

"Cut to the chase," Ira told him as he emerged on Forty-third Street, shielding the cellular phone as much as possible from the surrounding street noise. It would be up to Vida to carry the conversation from here.

"Ira, hunting me down has been a major goal in your life, just as hunting down serial killers has been in mine. You could argue that my methods have turned me into a serial killer. I'll grant you the point. Labels don't mean that much to me.

"But you must admit there is a major difference between me and those other serial murderers. The people I kill slaughter innocent people. Maybe that doesn't exactly make me blameless. I'm not in Mother Teresa's league, but I'm still a notch above Adolf Hitler or Saddam Hussein."

As he neared his quarry, Ira slipped the cellular phone into his pants pocket; he was going to need his good hand. Less than a hundred feet ahead, he could see a man's legs beneath a pay phone on the corner. The body language of the woman on the other phone said she was wrapping up her call. Ira drew his gun.

"All right, so you're not the scum of the earth. But you're still a wanted felon," said Vida.

"So is the Slasher. Isn't it your duty as law enforcement officers to stop his reign of terror, if you can?"

"He's not our case," answered Vida.

"If you had the chance to stop him, you wouldn't take it?"

"How about we cut the crap, David? You know we'd nab the Slasher even if it isn't our assignment."

"I'll bet you would. He's tearing this city apart. Race relations have never been New York's long suit. These killings are like throwing accelerant on a raging fire."

"Yes. Everyone's going crazy," snapped Vida. "Fringe white power groups are endorsing this lunatic's killing spree. Radical Hispanic leaders are calling for their people to arm themselves. Most black leaders are siding with mainstream Hispanic politicos, protesting the way the city is handling the matter. They figure, maybe rightly so, that they're next if the Slasher gets away with this shit. Everyone's calling for the mayor's resignation. This town is going to hell in a handcart. That about cover it?"

"Yes, that'll save us a lot of time."

Ira was less than twenty feet from the pay phone. Taking a deep breath, he moved to the right, ready to confront the fugitive he'd been hunting for over seven years.

"Are you trying to propose some kind of deal, David?"

"Yes."

"What happened, David? Did you run into a roadblock you can't get around on your own?"

Only his target's legs were in view. Two more short steps and Ira would be face to face with the perpetrator.

"Very perceptive on your part, Ms. Johnson."

One more step. Would Vandemark go for a gun?

"Okay, lay it out for me," Vida said. What was taking Ira so long? How much longer could she keep Vandemark occupied?

Ira took his final step, raised his weapon in a Weaver stance, and yelled, "Freeze!"

Everyone within earshot complied immediately.

Ira found himself covering a terrified, freckle-faced young man, who was gaping at him uncomprehendingly. "Sorry," Levitt muttered, "my mistake," then lowered his cannon and slipped it into his holster. Frantically searching the street for his quarry, Ira pulled out the cellular phone.

"There's a man who works for the federal government," explained David. "He's upper echelon, I believe. I think he's involved somehow in the Latino Family Murders, but I don't have any hard evidence yet. There's a good chance he's not the actual killer. The Slasher might be someone who works for him. The guy's got some heavy-duty muscle surrounding him."

There were no other pay phones on the street. Vandemark had to be on another cellular. But where? As Levitt searched the surrounding first- and second-floor windows, he heard Vida ask, "What do you want?"

"I need hard information on this character. I'm not getting anywhere with my usual sources. I can't penetrate the wall of classified security around the man. Maybe you can."

"I'm still waiting to hear what you're proposing, David."

A marked hesitation, then: "Here it is. I give you the name. You go after him. If you bag him and put him away, he's yours. But I stick around in the background, just to make sure you don't screw up. You understand me?"

"Clearly. But this doesn't change anything. If Ira and I get the chance to bust you, we will."

"I wouldn't have it any other way."

What in blue blazes was going on here? Ira wondered as he made his way along the street. Vandemark was willing to give up his prey to strike a deal. That certainly wasn't the David Vandemark he knew. Something had changed. But what?

"Who's the man?" asked Vida.

"Charles Camden."

Ira heard the name at the exact moment he spotted Vandemark at a table in the second-floor windowed dining area of a Wendy's.

"Are you completely nuts, Vandemark?" Ira said as he raced into the fast-food joint.

"Maybe a little," answered David. "Not enough to matter."

"Then are you kidding?" Ira switched the phone to his injured hand. The cast made it nearly impossible for Ira's stubby fingers to grasp it.

"No."

"You really don't know who Charles Camden is?" Ira drew his gun again and glanced up the staircase to the second floor.

"No. Why would I be talking to you if I did?"

"Don't you ever read anything in the papers besides the crime news?"

"What the hell's that supposed to mean?"

Ira's foot reached the first step. "It means that Charles Camden has been mentioned in connection with some pretty significant political stories several times over the past ten years."

"In what way?"

"He's been on the edge of some heavy CIA and NSC business that came to the press's attention," said Ira as he systematically climbed the stairs.

"The National Security Council?" David repeated in hushed tones.

"What else? So do you see now how off the mark you are thinking Camden's the Slasher?"

"I . . . How do you figure that, Ira?"

Ira reached the top of the stairs, which were at the back of the restaurant. Vandemark was up near the front. Probably right behind that damn stanchion by the window. Ira moved forward, past early lunchers trying to pretend they didn't see Ira's gun.

Vida picked up the slack. "Think for a minute, man. Camden's big. Why would someone like him have anything to do with killing Hispanic New Yorkers? This guy's used to playing on the international scene. Slashing up local Latinos is not his style."

On the other side of the stanchion, Ira steeled himself. Ready, set . . .

"It might be someone in his organization."

"Then we'll investigate that possibility," said Vida. "But you've got to understand that this is going to take time. I don't know what Camden's into these days. There might be a lot of interdepartmental red tape."

Ira leaped from behind the stanchion, dropping automatically into a two-handed firing stance.

There was no one to yell "Freeze!" to.

❦

Climbing the fire escape behind the building next door to Wendy's, David spoke into his cellular. "The Slasher is due to strike again within the week."

"We had a deal, David! We told you about Camden!" Vida reminded him.

"But you also admit you can't do anything about the Slasher before he does some more wet work."

Wearily sitting down at the table Vandemark had evacuated, Ira asked, "So where does that leave us?"

"I'm going to continue investigating Camden's outfit from my end. You see what you can do with your contacts. If I find out one of Camden's men is the killer, I'll call you. If you pull him in, everything's jake. But if you can't hold him, he's mine whether you like it or not. That's the deal, take it or leave it."

"One last thing, David," Ira said.

"What?"

"What's changed?"

Ira's answer was a dial tone.

❦

Too close, thought David as he disappeared into the sea of hungry New Yorkers in search of the perfect lunch.

If he hadn't spotted Ira racing toward Wendy's out of the corner of his eye, he'd be in custody right now. Even so, the danger didn't register immediately. David had been too absorbed in the cellular phone gag. So busy patting himself on the back that he damn near got his ass busted.

Ira was right that something had changed. Levitt sensed it somehow. It was David. He had lost his critical edge.

34

Vida sat in a chair by the window of Ira's hotel room, sipping a club soda with lime from room service. She overlooked Manhattan's spectacular skyline, but her ears were tuned to Ira's voice. She could tell that his telephone conversation with Charles Camden wasn't going at all the way her partner had hoped.

Vida's recollections of Camden were numerous, though all thirdhand. Around Washington's Beltway, Camden was a familiar but somewhat shadowy figure. He'd been a player for decades in a town that was infamous for professional cannibalism.

Vida remembered that Camden had been involved in an attempt to free the hostages at the American embassy in Iran using mercenaries. The Carter White House had caught wind of it and asked him to hold off until the military took a crack at it. Of course they blew it. Camden's plan never got off the ground again after that.

Before that, Camden was some kind of liaison officer to the CIA during the Ford administration, always popping up in the midst of some crisis in the Middle East or in South or Central America. Never one of the highly visible major players. Always doing stuff in the background—setting things up, making deals for which others could take the credit.

Then there were his days at the NSC during the early Reagan years. From then on everything about the man became classified. Even now, with Clinton in office, Camden was a key power broker within the intelligence community.

It'd taken Ira nearly a dozen calls to Washington to hunt up a number where Camden could be reached. Ira finally had to call the Bureau chief directly and tell him that Camden's life might be in danger, that recent information they'd uncovered revealed David Vandemark might be gunning for him. This got the chief's attention. It wouldn't do to have a VIP like Camden turn up dead and later have it leak that a senior FBI official had prior knowledge of this danger but failed to act.

Despite this it took another hour for the number to materialize. When he rang Ira back, the chief insisted he'd had to call in several favors. Levitt had better be on the money with this information. It wasn't a smart move to bother someone of Camden's caliber with unfounded rumors and speculation. Ira assured him that the tip was solid. The chief would see for himself as soon as he had Ira's written report. Ira failed to mention he hadn't figured out how to compose that report to prevent Vida and him from coming off like a couple of green rookies.

When Ira got off the horn with the chief, he showed Vida the number he'd copied down for Camden. There was no address, but the area code indicated Manhattan.

"You don't think Vandemark might be on to something?" she said. "Camden's in New York. But so are eight million other people. That doesn't make them all Slasher suspects."

Ira nodded his agreement. "The thing is, we have solid evidence that each of Vandemark's victims was indeed a serial murderer. Even that coke dealer in Sanibel was wanted for questioning in the death of two DEA agents. Vandemark's got a perfect record so far. It's hard to argue with that kind of success."

"What d'you want to do about it?"

"We've got to warn Camden about Vandemark, of course. But I think we've also got to inform Camden about Vandemark's suspicion that the Slasher might be one of his men. Maybe Camden will let the Bureau discreetly investigate his personnel."

"And if he doesn't?"

"Let's cross that bridge if and when we come to it. Meanwhile I'm going to give Camden a ring."

The call to Camden had been going on for nearly twenty minutes, with Vida listening in on Ira's end. What she'd heard didn't sound promising.

When Ira hung up, he sat there for a long moment, staring at the silent phone. Vida knew he was processing information and would return to the real world as soon as he'd sorted through his impressions. As she waited, Vida suspected that she probably wouldn't like the conclusions her partner was reaching concerning Charles Camden.

When Ira got up and reached for his diet soda, which had been growing warm while he was on the phone, Vida asked, "Well, what did he say?"

"Thanks, but no thanks. He'll investigate Vandemark's suspicions using his own security personnel. The project he's involved with is too sensitive to allow any outsiders to even know its location."

"A pretty standard bureaucratic response. Did you expect anything different?"

"Not really."

"Then what's bothering you?"

"Charles Camden."

Vida let that hang in the air for a while. This was what she had feared. The knot in the pit of her stomach tightened, and she felt cold. Ira didn't need to say another word. She knew what he was thinking, and she didn't like it one bit. Still, she made herself ask, "What about Charles Camden?"

"He reacted all wrong. I expected him to balk at letting us check out his people. That's standard government operating procedure. But how would you think someone would react when he heard that a man who had already killed twenty people might be stalking him?"

"I suppose a person would be shocked. Maybe a little scared. Wasn't Camden?"

"Not a bit."

"Was he trying to be macho?"

"No. In fact, he sounded relieved. Isn't that nuts? And you know what else? He didn't react much when I told him the reason Vandemark was checking him out. Camden had absolutely no interest in why some lunatic might think he was involved in the Latino Family Murders. I think that's pretty peculiar."

Vida fidgeted uncomfortably in her seat, not wanting this talk to continue but unable to find a way to stop it. "Well, Ira, the man is an important executive. Maybe he didn't want to be bothered with a lot of details. That's how some of those high-powered types are."

Ira scowled at Vida. "Executives don't want to be bothered about inconsequential details. I was telling the man his life was in danger, and he didn't even want to know why!"

"Maybe he's had death threats before?"

"That's possible. But most death threats come from anonymous people, usually cranks and losers who couldn't hurt a fly even if they really wanted to. I was informing Camden that a known killer might be after him. All he asked was that I send a copy of Vandemark's file to his Washington office. It doesn't make sense."

"But that way it'd take the file at least a couple days to reach him! That's being pretty cool."

"Too cool by half, if you ask me."

"Meaning?"

"There's only one reason Camden wouldn't be anxious to get all the information on Vandemark he could get his hands on. And that's because he's already got a line on our boy."

"How?"

"I don't know. But Camden hobnobs with presidents. A guy like that has got better connections than the FBI and the CIA put together."

Vida got up from her chair, turned her back to Ira, and stared distractedly out the window. "Then there's a good chance Camden may do our job for us?"

"Maybe. But it's the way Camden might do it that worries me."

"Are you suggesting that Charles Camden would use excessive force in dealing with Vandemark?"

"That's a delicate way of putting it. Come to think of it, I seem to recall that Camden's name came up a few times while the Carter administration was investigating the CIA's alleged assassination of South American political leaders. He walked away clean. No charges were leveled against him."

Vida turned around. "Careful, Ira, you're beginning to sound like a liberal." Her joke lay in the silence like a dead thing.

Ira took a deep breath and shrugged. He picked up his soda and walked over to join her at the window. "You think I should forget all about it, don't you?" he said.

"Yes. Camden's one of the biggest power brokers in Capitol Hill's inner circle. Jesus, Ira, think of what you're suggesting! Remember, I only crossed a junior member of that club once, and I ended up in Siberia working with you on a case no one else wants to touch."

"And you figure with someone like Camden it could get worse?"

"Damn straight."

"I guess you're right."

"Ira, I like you. You're the best person I've met at the Bureau. But I need this job. I've got a mother and three brothers who depend on me. I can't afford to get involved in a political scandal."

Ira walked over to the bed and sat down heavily. On the way he'd pulled out his wallet. He flipped it open and looked at his Bureau ID. Vida watched in silence, wishing it were over.

In a voice that was barely audible, Ira said, "I joined the Bureau when I was a young man, back when I still suffered from the delusion that police work had something to do with justice. You'd think that twenty-eight years on the job would have cured me of that. I guess it did. After a while I realized justice was nothing more than an intellectual concept. The reality is that you and I work for a monstrous machine. Its purpose, supposedly, is to mete out justice. But that's not what it actually does. It only enforces laws. And sometimes the laws are wrong. That's not supposed to make any difference, though. We're law enforcement officers.

"Along the way I learned there were different ways to interpret the law. One set of rules applies to the rich and connected. Another, stricter set of laws applies to the poor.

"Then I discovered the machine could be used against its own. Every morning I return to that basement office reminds me of that fact. What I'm saying is that I know the score. I'm no fool. It'd be crazy to buck Camden. It'd be suicidal."

Vida came over and sat on the other twin bed, directly across from Ira. "Then that means you're going to be sensible?"

"No, that means *you* are. Whatever I do, I'm doing on my own. Alone."

"But Ira, why?"

The giant rolled over onto the narrow bed. "Because I'm old, ugly, and stupid. And because I talked to a younger man today who's putting everything on the line to save another family from being murdered in a few days. Maybe he's crazy. I don't know. But what he's doing isn't crazy. If I don't help him stop these killings I'm not going to be able to live with myself."

Vida sat staring at her partner as if she were seeing him

for the first time. She knew he was right, of course, but she also knew something else.

"Don't turn into Don Quixote on me," she said. "There are fights you can't win, Ira. Hell, you don't even know for sure that Camden's involved. Think about it. Please."

Ira closed his eyes. "I'm tired of playing at dealing out justice. It's time I took a chance on the real thing."

"What does that mean?"

"Maybe you'll figure it out someday, Vida. I'm too tired to explain it right now. I'm going to catch a nap. I'll see you at dinner."

Having been dismissed, Vida stood up and walked to the door. She stood there for a moment trying to think of something to say. Their partnership had gone sour so suddenly. Vida didn't want to leave things the way they were between Ira and her.

But Ira had chosen a path that Vida couldn't follow. He was alone in the world with responsibility for no one but himself. He could afford his heroic fantasy. Besides why should she watch her career go down the drain? Let Camden and Vandemark kill each other off. It'd probably be a better world without them. Too bad Ira Levitt had decided to sacrifice his life along with theirs.

Vida opened the door and stepped into the hallway. As she made her way back to her room, the exchange with Ira kept haunting her.

"I'm tired of playing at dealing out justice. It's time I took a chance on the real thing."

"What does that mean?"

"Maybe you'll figure it out someday, Vida."

35

Charles Camden felt incredibly relieved. At last he knew who the spy was.

Until Agent Levitt called, the spy's identity had been a looming question mark. But Camden no longer had to worry that the FBI, CIA, local police, newspapers, or anyone else important had discovered the real purpose of his West Side installation. The spy was a psychotic, with no ties to anyone. A nonentity. David Vandemark was a vigilante, interested only in tracking down the Latino Family Killer. The fool had no idea of the magnitude of the affair he had blundered into. Well, that ignorance would soon be dealt with. Permanently.

Twenty minutes before Levitt phoned, Camden had received a call from McGuire and Hanson. They said David Vandemark had returned to the van for a change of clothing. He left the garage carrying a personal computer and a metal case. Camden's men followed him to a fifth-floor apartment on Twenty-seventh Street. The subject remained there for some forty-five minutes, then left. Hanson and McGuire decided to let him go on his way without a tail. Why bother? After all, they'd already discovered what they were after. They had tracked him to his lair.

Inquiries revealed the apartment belonged to Angela Quinoñes, a surviving relative of the first victims of the Latino Family Killer.

Hanson and McGuire had surreptitiously entered the Quinoñes apartment. Both were skilled at breaking and entering, and Camden felt confident they'd left behind no evidence of their visit.

Once inside, they had used five rolls of film to record the apartment's physical layout. While Hanson shot the interior from almost every angle imaginable, McGuire drafted a detailed floor plan of the apartment that included every stick of furniture, every appliance, closet, and doorway. Distances were measured with a tape measure and jotted down.

They'd delivered their findings to Charles Camden less than an hour ago. McGuire's floor plan was taped to the wall, and eight-by-ten glossies were spread across Camden's desk.

Everything in Charles Camden's universe was in order once more.

The Latino Family Killer's original time schedule was again in place. *No hay problema.* But there would be one amendment to the original plan. Instead of only striking three more times, the Slasher would claim four more sets of victims.

The Alfredo Martinez and Esteban Moreno families would have been perfect candidates for the Slasher, but neither family would be murdered this weekend, as originally planned.

The Slasher was going to change his pattern somewhat.

On his first outing, the Latino Family Killer had missed a member of the Quinoñes family. The tabloids were going to love this. Camden could just imagine the sleazy, voyeuristic fun they'd have speculating as to why the Slasher had returned to slaughter Angela Quinoñes, the only surviving member of the ill-fated Quinoñes clan.

But that was nothing compared to the field day they would have once it was discovered that the man who died with Angela Quinoñes was a wanted murderer himself.

Yes, everything was working out neatly. Within the sanctuary of his pristine office Charles Camden smiled broadly. There was great contentment in that smile.

36

David Vandemark was getting impatient. He'd been hiding behind the Dumpster for nearly two hours.

The cellular phone episode with Ira Levitt and Vida had gone wrong. He'd planned to lay out everything he'd learned so far, being careful not to reveal that he'd acquired most of the information telepathically. He'd hoped that by mapping out his investigation in a professional manner, he would pique Levitt's interest sufficiently to go after the Slasher. David needed Ira's help, and he also wanted to get the agent off his back for a while.

But when the time came, David had jettisoned his plan and then antagonized both Levitt and Johnson without giving them any real details about his investigation. Splendid. And what about that preposterous deal he proposed? David couldn't believe he'd actually offered to walk away and let the FBI handle the Latino Family Killer case. What had he been thinking?

If Levitt could handle Camden, would he really abandon the hunt? Would he allow the FBI to merely lock the Slasher away? Would he let the Latino Family Murderer live?

To David's amazement, the answer to all those questions was a resounding and unqualified yes.

And the reason for this sudden reversal of all his patterns, his stated intentions, his *mission*? Angela.

It was increasingly evident that her introduction into his life was prompting some unforeseen and unaccustomed changes. First there was the passion. Then the reemergence of the old David Vandemark. And now? An uncontrollable urge to retire, spurred on by what? Love? Yes, David had to admit that Angela Quinoñes had wreaked gentle, stealthy havoc on his status quo.

Seven years of hunting crazed murderers and sending them to their just reward.

Seven years was plenty of time for a person to burn out on any type of work. It was a wonder he had lasted this long. Alone. Always in danger. Always on the move. Looking back, it seemed like someone else's life. But it wasn't. David couldn't allow himself that comforting fiction. There'd already been enough of that kind of denial.

So as he sat hiding behind a trash bin in a filthy alley, David wondered idly what this all meant in terms of his future.

It was painfully apparent to him that Levitt wouldn't be able to handle Camden. Not even a federal cop had the muscle to take on someone with Camden's connections. A case like this could drag on for years through legal channels without ever reaching a satisfactory conclusion.

After going 'round and 'round with it, David realized he was stuck with this case. It wasn't only dreams of an early retirement that prompted his desire to be free of it. Right from the start this job hadn't felt right. To begin with, this was New York, a town that had never been anything but trouble for him. Then there was his meeting Angela. As pleasantly as that had turned out, encountering someone whose mind he couldn't read should have warned David off. It was a bad omen. Then Levitt had showed up in town. And on top of it all, David's chief suspect was a White House insider.

Everything that could go wrong had gone wrong. It was time to cut and run, to hop into the van with Angela and head upstate. Angela would probably love Willow, New York.

But if he did that, another innocent Hispanic family would die in the next week or so. David knew Levitt wouldn't be able to cut it. He was trapped in a mire of red tape and regulations.

The ball was back in David's court. Would he be able to run with it?

On that count David wasn't at all sure. This time his qualms didn't feel like just a new lover's sudden selfishness and caution surrounding his own mortality. The rock-hard pit in his stomach warned him that things were out of control, and there was a better than even chance that he might not survive this hunt.

❧❧❧

Movement in front of the warehouse stirred David from his dark introspection. He'd been hiding four blocks from Camden's installation, waiting for someone who might shed light on Camden's activities. He hoped at this distance he'd be out of range of the surveillance cameras. He couldn't think of a way to pinpoint the location of all of Camden's spy cameras without being spotted. Distance from the installation was his only defense. So he'd been keeping an eye on the place with his high-powered binoculars.

Thus far, this scheme hadn't worked either. Five people had left the installation since David's arrival. Three of them had gotten into waiting cars, making them useless for David's purposes. The other two had walked off downtown, away from where David was lurking.

David had stashed the binoculars behind the Dumpster and taken off after both of the pedestrians. This hadn't been easy because he'd had to sprint at least three blocks out of his way to avoid detection. By the time he caught up with his quarry he was drenched in sweat and panting like a racehorse after a half-mile stretch at Belmont. That indignity wouldn't have been so hard to accept if both pedestrians hadn't entered different garages and then driven off in private cars. Both times David trudged back to his hiding place, muttering to himself that more people in this city should use mass transit.

Suddenly it looked as if David's luck might be changing. A man had come out of the warehouse and was walking in his direction. He was in his late thirties, slim, with curly dark hair and wire-rimmed glasses, carrying a briefcase.

David ditched the binoculars and followed his quarry, who had turned a corner.

❧❧❧

Chester Pinyon was on duty at the video monitors. He was grooming his fingernails with a tiny screwdriver he carried in a pocket pen holder. The screwdriver came in handy for minor repairs and adjustments on the video console. He wasn't a video technician, but he knew enough to correct a flopping screen or an off-color image. Besides, such repairs broke up the tedium. After yesterday's excitement Chester was finding it hard to settle into his usual alpha state. He was afraid he might miss something important on the screens. Chester knew something was up. When that bum showed up yesterday a person could have cut the tension in this room with a knife. The bum had worried Mr. Camden. And anything that worried Mr. Camden scared the bejesus out of Chester. So he had decided to remain exceptionally vigilant today.

So far, his diligence had rewarded him with nothing but boredom. This had been just another dreadfully dull day at the installation. Thank God he only had another hour left on this shift.

On one of the screens Chester watched Herbert Shelley leave through the warehouse's front entrance. Looked like the man had decided to take off early today. Shelley worked in the high-security area of the installation. Chester didn't know Shelley very well, having only met him in the coffee room once or twice. But he'd watched the man come and go from work every weekday for the past eighteen months. Chester thought about how odd it was to see so much of someone and not know anything about him, other than the fact that Shelley was one of the few people here who walked to work and that he was some kind of a doctor. His security file card listed the man as Dr. Herbert Shelley.

With nothing else to do, Chester followed Herbert Shelley's progress from one monitor to the next. His interest began to wane when Shelley faded into the distance of monitor sixteen, the surveillance net's farthest camera. Chester was about to turn away from the screen when someone jogged into view on it. Chester instantly recognized the lone runner. He'd been instructed to stay on the alert for him.

Chester punched the red button on his intercom. A second or two later Charles Camden's voice came on the line. "Yes?"

"He's back sir. Heading east from camera sixteen. Looks like he's tailing Herbert Shelley."

"Thank you, Chester. Now clear the line."

❦

Charles Camden pressed another button on his intercom. A man's voice answered, "Garage."

In a clear, well-modulated voice, Camden said, "The target's heading east on Seventeenth, following Herbert Shelley. Remove Shelley from the scene before acting on Vandemark."

"On our way" was the only response Charles Camden received. The line went dead.

Camden stood up and headed for the security control room. He was glad he had set up this alternate plan in case Vandemark showed up at the installation. It wasn't quite as satisfying as having this pest become one of the Latino Family Killer's victims, but it would do. David Vandemark was about to become a New York City mugging statistic. Perhaps it was for the best. The sooner Vandemark was eliminated as a possible threat, the sooner operations could return to normal. No reason to take needless chances with this lunatic.

❦

On the south side of the warehouse, a loading bay opened. Three cars drove out through it, one of them a cab. They turned onto the side street, heading east.

❦

David was less than a half block behind Herbert Shelley. He wasn't worried about losing the man. Shelley was enjoying his walk home from work, savoring this marvelous day, completely unaware of being followed.

David hoped to get a reading on this fellow, learn some pertinent facts about him and then use them to telepathically pry loose the information he needed. This way David could interrogate the man without his ever being aware of what was going on.

To do this, he needed an object of Shelley's from which to get a deep reading, something the man had been carrying on his person for a while. David considered knocking the guy's briefcase out of his hand and scanning it quickly while he picked it up, but his quarry might think he was trying to steal the case. David didn't want the guy agitated, since it was easier to pick a man's brain if he remained calm.

The problem abruptly solved itself. Herbert Shelley stopped at a newsstand to pick up a paper. David watched him dip into his pocket for change. The change might do the trick. The coins had probably been in his pocket all day, maybe even two days. That might be long enough for them to have picked up a solid imprint.

David quickly fished a dollar bill out of his pocket and paid the newsstand vendor for a paper. He received four coins in change. He picked up the coins from the counter one at a time.

The first, a quarter, had last been in the possession of a woman. David quickly dropped it into his pants pocket.

No reading on the second, a dime. Into the pocket.

The nickel had traces of a policeman and a waitress on it. No good.

A teenage boy had used a second dime to purchase a girlie magazine.

David saw his quarry up the street, disappearing among the thick throng of passersby. Turning back to the newsstand, he picked up a Three Musketeers bar and fished out another dollar bill.

The man behind the counter looked at the bill and said, "How about paying for this with the change I gave you? I'm getting kind of low."

"Need it for the bus," David explained as he squinted, trying to spot Herbert Shelley.

The vendor plunked down the change—one dime, one quarter.

David snatched them up and knew instantly that he had what he was after. He turned and ran down the street after the man he now knew to be Herbert Shelley, a psychiatrist with an associate's degree in biochemistry. He'd graduated from Harvard Medical School and lived on West Seventy-first Street near Central Park. A psychiatrist? Interesting . . .

As David trotted off, he heard the vendor calling after him. "Hey mac! You forgot your candy bar and paper!"

❦

David spotted Herbert Shelley casually strolling along the street. He'd have no trouble catching up to him at a street corner and starting a conversation. "Say, aren't you Herb Shelley? We went to Harvard Medical together. Don't you remember me?" From there David would steer the talk to where Shelley would be forced to think about his work. He would lie about what he was doing for a living, but his mind would be telling David the truth.

To David's horror, a car pulled up to the curb beside Herbert Shelley, and the driver called the doctor's name. David watched an expression of recognition register on Herbert's face. The driver signaled Shelley to get into the car, and the man obliged. Damn! Why did everything go wrong with this case?

The car started to pull away from the curb. David looked around for some way to follow it. Directly across the street was a cab whose passenger was getting out. David sprinted toward it. The departing passenger saw him coming and held the door for him. That old David Vandemark luck was turning around, heading in the right direction for a change.

David hopped into the rear seat and said to the driver, "You're not going to believe this, but I want you to—"

The driver turned in his seat and pointed a gun at David. There wasn't the usual partition separating the front seat from the back. The man with the gun smiled and said, "No, pal, *you're* not going to believe *this*."

David's arm lashed out, backhanding the bridge of the driver's nose. The gun slipped from the stunned man's hand and fell to the floor at David's feet. He was reaching down for it when something looped over his head and around his neck. Before he could react, he found himself being dragged toward the door and nearly out the window. His hands clawed at the wire digging into his neck

A garrote!

A quick telepathic probe informed David that his attacker was the man who'd held the door open for him. He should've known such courtesy in New York had to have an ulterior motive. Through his rapidly blurring vision, he noticed another car screech to a halt across the street. A man jumped out and was running his way.

It hardly seemed important at the moment. David knew he'd be dead in another thirty seconds or so if he didn't free himself from this garrote. Frantically monitoring his attacker's thoughts, David learned that the man was uncomfortable about the work he was doing. Garroting David had been a desperate act when he saw him backhand the driver. The killer was off-balance. With the world turning into a burning red blur, David waited patiently for the killer to shift his footing. As soon as he sensed the move beginning David reached behind his head and grabbed the startled assassin's wrists. He then threw himself forward with everything he had. This effort was rewarded with the sound of teeth shattering against the roof of the cab.

Without bothering to tear the loosened garrote from his neck, David again backhanded the driver, who had been reaching over the seat to retrieve his gun.

Turning around, David saw the third man reach inside

his sport jacket. David grabbed the gun off the floor of the cab and shot him. The bullet caught the man in the shoulder and spun him around. He crashed to the pavement.

David pulled the garrote from his neck, feeling it tear loose from the flesh it had dug itself into. When he turned around to inspect the garrote's owner, David saw his stunned attacker holding one hand to his ruined mouth, blood dripping between the fingers. The garrote trailed out of a bracelet affair on the man's other wrist. So David gave the wire another hard tug. The killer again bounced off the door and disappeared from view.

Still holding the driver's gun, David stepped out on the street side of the car. The man he'd pumped a bullet into was on his hands and knees, trying to reach his weapon. David kicked him in the face and ran across the street. The crowd of startled onlookers parted to let him pass. No one was going to try to stop this frightening-looking man with the smoking gun, bloody neck, and fiery eyes.

37

Forty minutes later Charles Camden had been fully briefed on the incident. The operative who had whisked Herbert Shelley away had dropped the psychiatrist off at his West Side apartment. On the way back to the installation he decided to see if anything was still happening where the hit went down. He wasn't sure if his partners were going to leave Vandemark's body there or dump it elsewhere. The operative figured he was in no danger driving past. He hadn't been involved in the killing. No witness could finger him.

He was extremely surprised to find his three colleagues on the scene, along with two squad cars and an ambulance. The operative parked down the street and discreetly walked back to where everyone was gathered. Standing on the sidelines amid a gathering crowd, he was able to piece together what had happened.

His associates told the police that someone had tried to rob the cabbie. A Good Samaritan walking by on the street had tried to intervene. Most of his teeth had been knocked out for his trouble. Of course, the Good Samaritan had dropped his garrote down a storm drain by the time the police arrived.

The third man, who had been shot on the street, was unconscious and so couldn't tell his part of the tale. Along with the bullet hole in his shoulder, it appeared that this poor guy had a broken jaw. The police found a permit in the unconscious man's wallet for the gun witnesses said was his. The cops were guessing that he'd tried to stop the robbery and caught a slug as his reward. They would sort it out later. Right now everybody—including the cabbie who had a broken nose—had to get to the hospital.

◆◆◆◆

Camden was surprised by this turn of events. Who would have thought that psycho could prove to be so formidable? The men Vandemark had taken down were all pros. They weren't the best money could buy, but they should have been able to handle Vandemark without working up a sweat. This Fruit Loop was a hell of a lot tougher than anyone had realized.

Camden reached for a cigar and sat back to contemplate what this revised assessment of David Vandemark would mean to the operation. He decided that not much in his original plans need be altered. David Vandemark and Angela Quiñones would still become Slasher victims, the Latino Family Killer would strike one night earlier— tomorrow night—and the Slasher wouldn't enter the victims' premises alone. As an added safety precaution, McGuire and Hanson would accompany him into the Quiñones apartment.

Blowing smoke into the air, Camden thought—with

some relief—that at least his men had gotten Herbert Shelley out of the area before the fireworks went off. Dr. Shelley would have been upset by that kind of violence. Herbert could stomach death only as long as it remained an abstract concept, far removed from his reality. Camden didn't like the man's hypocritical morality and squeamishness.

But Camden needed Shelley to control the Slasher. Without that control the entire operation would quickly unravel. He thought momentarily about sending a couple of his men over to keep an eye on Shelley but changed his mind. He reasoned that Vandemark had chosen Shelley by accident, without realizing what an important component he was in Camden's scheme. No reason to push the panic button prematurely. That psycho had simply followed the first person who walked out of the installation. He had probably hoped to pump Shelley for information. Sending someone to guard Shelley would only spook the man.

For tonight Dr. Herbert Shelley would be secure in the sanctuary of his own home. Vandemark could have no idea where Dr. Shelley lived. In fact it was impossible for him to even know Shelley's name. If Vandemark did have that information, the good doctor would still remain safe behind his unlisted phone number. Even his apartment was rented under an assumed name, as an added precaution.

Still, it might be a good idea to have one of the boys escort Shelley to work tomorrow morning. Camden doubted that Vandemark would come anywhere near the installation again, but one could never tell with a head case.

38

David Vandemark was angry with the world in general and with Charles Camden in particular for sending hired killers after him. And he was mad at Ira Levitt and Vida Johnson for not doing their job. And annoyed with Angela Quiñones for not having bandages in her apartment. He was angry with everyone, in fact, including himself.

He berated himself for having walked into such a blatant trap. Why hadn't he scanned the cabbie and passenger before getting into that too-convenient taxi? He'd been concentrating on the car driving off with Herbert Shelley, but that was no excuse. He was lucky to have come out of that fiasco alive, he thought with sullen fury.

Things kept getting stranger and stranger. How was it that he had set off to stalk one lone psychotic killer and now found himself fighting off a whole gang of paid assassins? That was exactly what those guys were. They were professional hit men in the employ of Charles Camden. David had unearthed this information by reading the cabbie's gun.

Unfortunately, the driver didn't know exactly what was going on at Camden's hideaway. Camden's organization was divided in such a way that there was no communication between departments. The security people had no idea that some employees at Sal Taglia Enterprises were hired guns. And neither group knew what went on in the heart of the installation, where the eggheads worked. Dr. Shelley was the chief egghead. But the cabbie and the other hired guns had no idea of the nature of Shelley's work. It seemed no one except Camden knew all of the players.

The more pieces of this puzzle David turned up, the less sense it all made.

❦

David went to his van for a first aid kit and a lightweight turtleneck sweater to replace his blood-spattered shirt. The sweater would hide his injuries when he went out later.

Back at Angela's apartment, he cleaned and disinfected his neck wound. Not an easy job. Very painful. The wire had cut deep. Any deeper and it would have gotten the jugular. Too close. Much too close.

David decided it was time to change his strategy. Until now he had been keeping a low profile, nosing around on the sly, trying to pick up scraps of information without revealing his presence. He'd failed miserably on that last count. Camden knew he was on his trail. And he'd sent a goon squad out to kill David. With the stakes escalating and the rules being tossed out the window, that made it a whole new game.

He felt good about this. It meant he could stop pussyfooting around and get down and dirty; he liked that much better. There was a nice vendetta-like honesty about it. David had to assume that everyone involved with Camden was part of some complex plot. That sounded paranoid, but the evidence pointed in that direction. After all, even paranoids had enemies. Crazy or not, there didn't seem to be any other conclusion.

That decided it. From this point on, David would act as if the people he encountered were out to get him. He would treat them accordingly: shoot first and ask questions later.

Unfortunately for Herbert Shelley, he was the next person David planned to encounter.

39

Herbert Shelley had an irresistible desire for some Häagen-Dazs strawberry ice cream.

After Jim Barkely, that nice man from the installation, gave him a ride home Herbert had done a long-overdue load of laundry and then eaten a solitary dinner at a neighborhood restaurant. Herbert hated eating alone, but he had been doing so quite often since his wife left him. Six months ago Maggie Shelley had decided she'd had enough of Herbert's uncommunicative brooding and high-and-mighty attitude. Their four-year union had produced no offspring, so Maggie just packed up one morning and took off for California, leaving a note of explanation on the kitchen table. Herbert didn't care. The stimulation he was getting from his work was all he needed these days. Maggie had become a burden with her constant emotional and sexual demands. Herbert felt lucky to be rid of her.

After dinner Dr. Herbert Shelley returned to his two-bedroom apartment to read through a couple of articles in this month's *New England Journal of Medicine*. He thought they might relate to the work he was doing at the installation. He was somewhat disappointed, though not surprised, to discover they didn't. He and his assistant, Dr. James Hoover, were the only people farsighted enough to grasp the endless possibilities that awaited them along the avenue of research they were presently pioneering.

The ice cream urge hit at about eight o'clock. Herbert could feel that sweet delight tickling his taste buds. There was a deli two blocks over that carried Häagen-Dazs. And if they didn't have strawberry, the convenience store on the next block would. This craving would not be denied. Herbert had to have his late-night treat. The evening would be ruined without it. So he threw on his sport coat and went off in search of frozen taste sensations.

On his way out through the lobby Herbert waved good-naturedly to Buddy, the huge black doorman. Herb always felt secure knowing Buddy was standing guard at the front gate of the castle, ready to fend off burglars, rapists, and the odd Jehovah's Witness or two.

When he got outside Herbert was so intent on his quest that he didn't notice the man approaching him until the stranger said, "Well, I'll be damned! It is you! Herb Shelley! How you doing, pal?"

Shelley turned around to look at the man who'd called his name. Herbert was quite good at remembering faces, but he was drawing a blank on this one. Maybe the Vandyke was throwing him off. Giving up, Herbert said, "I'm sorry. Do I know you?"

The stranger smiled warmly and said, "I'm hurt, Herbie. You don't remember. But I guess I can understand that. How about I give you a little hint, to jog your memory?"

Then the man with the Vandyke kicked him in the balls.

Herbert Shelley doubled over as a wave of pain and nausea washed over him. But before he could hit the ground the stranger had grabbed his shoulders and straightened him up. He couldn't resist this aid. The man was very strong. But it wasn't only his aching scrotum that kept him from fighting back. Herbert thought he finally recognized the stranger. It had to be Billy Weston, the bully who had done the same thing to him back in sixth grade. No one else could be that low.

Herbert was aware that he was walking with the stranger's help. When he recovered somewhat, he realized uneasily that the man was leading him into Central Park. Herb tried in vain to struggle free from his tormentor.

Something hard was jammed into his belly. Herbert looked down. In the park's dim light he could see the something was a gun with a silencer. *Oh my God! I'm being mugged!*

"No, you're not," said the stranger. "We're going off to have a nice long talk. That's what old friends do when they haven't seen each other for a while."

"Billy?" Herbert asked in a quavering voice.

"No, my name's David Vandemark."

"But I don't know any David Vandemark."

"You do now," David said as he shoved Dr. Shelley behind a clump of bushes and followed him. Herb bounced against a stone wall and hit the ground. When he had struggled into a sitting position, a menacing-looking gun was pointed directly between his eyes.

Smiling, David said, "Your boss tried to have me killed this afternoon."

"I have no idea what you're talking about! Who do you—"

"I'm talking about Charles Camden, the man you work for. I want you to tell me about your job, Herbie."

This shut him up. As scary as this man was, Herbert didn't yet fear him as much as he did Camden. No matter what this wretched man did to him, Herbert resolved to never reveal anything about Project Jack.

"Yes, tell me about Project Jack."

Herbert stared at his captor in utter bewilderment. *How could this man know about Project Jack? Only ten people in the whole country are supposed to be aware of the project's existence.*

The smiling man asked, "Who are those ten people?"

Unable to stop himself, Herbert Shelley mentally listed the entire roll call of those in the know. *How does this man know about the ten insiders on the project? What else has he uncovered? He can't possibly know the project's purpose, could he?*

"Not yet, but you're going to tell me all about it," said the stranger as he poked Herbert in the forehead with his gun.

Being an individual of above-average intelligence, Herb soon figured out what was going on. *My God! He's reading my mind! It's not possible!*

"Ah, but it is, Herbie. I'm sure it's a shock to someone in your particular profession. But that's exactly what I'm doing."

He'll find out about the Latino Family Murders! Everyone will find out about Project Jack!

"Don't you think people have a right to know, Herb? You and your playmates have been bad boys. Twenty-four people are dead. And it's your fault."

Twenty-four? Then he doesn't know about Atlanta!

"I do now."

And so it went, David saying things to spur Dr. Shelley's thoughts, then reading his involuntary mental responses. Almost like tapping a knee with a reflex hammer. Each exchange revealed more of the story. At first David played with his captive, jokingly prodding the psychiatrist onward. But as more facts came out, Vandemark lost his sense of humor. His questions slowly changed into angrily whispered demands. The truth was more dreadful than he had suspected. Shelley's fear of David began to override his awe of Charles Camden. For a while the answers flowed freely from Dr. Shelley's mind.

But then the doctor realized he was thinking himself into a possible life sentence at Sing Sing. He tried to cloak his thoughts by chanting nursery rhymes in his head. David put an end to that by slamming a fist into Dr. Shelley's face, knocking out two teeth. There was no more chanting.

It occurred to Dr. Shelley that a prison term was the least of his worries. This crazed man with the blazing eyes and the power to read thoughts was quite capable of killing him. Herbert decided he would do anything to keep this monstrous person happy. He started to tell his captor everything he wanted to know vocally, without further prompting.

David sat back on his haunches, listening to Shelley's tale unwind. The doctor told him of his early research in college, which the board of trustees had eventually banned. He related how, years later, Charles Camden had approached him to head up a research project. Camden had read some of Shelley's college papers and was favorably impressed with them.

Shelley told about the first experiment, which had failed because they hadn't taken into account the setting and all the economic considerations. But the New York City test run had been carefully planned and was going perfectly. Shelley's pride in his work began to overcome his good sense. It became apparent to David that the man was actually bragging about his accomplishments. He believed that his work had a noble purpose. The dead didn't matter. They had been sacrificed to expand man's knowledge of himself. He knew Charles Camden had his own less lofty reasons for sponsoring the research, but as far as Herbert was concerned, it was being done in the sacred name of science.

Then David had the doctor tell him everything he knew about the installation. David listened without comment. He didn't let his face register the hatred he felt for Dr. Shelley and his associates. Until now Vandemark had allowed himself to believe that he'd already seen mankind at its lowest. He was learning how terribly mistaken he'd been in that assumption.

The other killers he had hunted were sick, twisted individuals who had let their sexual fantasies or delusions lead them to commit terrible crimes. They couldn't be allowed to live, but David viewed them as victims of their own madness. He had seen this clearly within their minds before he killed them.

But Charles Camden, Herbert Shelley, and the others at Taglia Enterprises were not insane. They were coolly rational men who knew exactly what they were doing. Their problem was that they had absolutely no sense of morality.

For them the end always justified the means. They held positions of responsibility and power, and maybe their power had confused them into believing that might equaled right. After all, the short-term goal was all that mattered these days. The consequences of their actions didn't concern them in the least, so long as they could avoid any accountability for them. These men were simply products of a society that demanded success before all else. People didn't count. Only results did.

David looked at Herbert, who was still spilling his guts. Tears rolled down the psychiatrist's face, blood dripped from his injured mouth. And David was filled with an overwhelming feeling of disgust for the doctor and his friends. Looking into Shelley's mind, he could see that the man's tears were not for what he had done. Shelley was crying because he'd been caught.

Shelley came to the end of his confession. He couldn't think of anything more to add. Neither could David. He'd heard more than enough. So he shot Herbert Shelley in the face. The mercury-tipped bullet blew out the back of the doctor's head. David got up and walked off. Someone would find the body in a day or two, when it started to smell.

As he stepped out onto Central Park West, David remembered his promise to Ira that he wouldn't kill the Slasher when he discovered his identity. Herbert Shelley hadn't been the actual Slasher, so killing him didn't violate that promise. But Shelley had been partly responsible for the Slasher's actions, so killing him had been just.

Unfortunately, the job wasn't complete. Herbert Shelley's death wouldn't end the Slasher's murder spree. The Latino Family Killer and his handlers had to be stopped before they struck again. But David realized that he couldn't accomplish that task alone. He needed help. And he knew exactly where to find it.

40

Dinner had been no fun at all for Ira Levitt. He and Vida had exchanged strained small talk throughout the meal. When dessert came, Ira informed his partner that she would have to act as the sole Bureau liaison to the NYPD for the rest of their stay in New York. This would free up Ira's time to continue the investigation in his own manner. Both knew what this meant, but neither commented on it.

Vida escaped to her room after dinner, and Ira wandered over to a dumpy Irish bar on Sixth Avenue for a couple of drinks. The gin and tonics did nothing to improve his disposition, but they did help him drift right off to sleep when he returned to his hotel. There was no all-night staring at the boob tube while he wrestled with his conscience. He had anesthetized his doubts and worries so he could get some rest. He would need his wits and energy tomorrow.

But this cure wasn't foolproof. If quality rather than quantity is the true measure of a thing, then you might even say this remedy sort of backfired. Ira's sleep was plagued by dreams of bureaucrats in the White House carrying bloody butcher knives. The dreams were interrupted before they became too horrific. Interrupted by a sound: something scratching on metal, then a distinctly metallic click.

Someone was picking the lock on Ira's hotel room door.

Ira reached under his pillow and pulled out his gun. He then rose and tiptoed to the door. Might as well yank it open and greet his visitor. There was much to be said for the element of surprise.

As Ira's hand closed around the knob, the door flew open and slammed into his jaw. Levitt's world exploded in a Fourth of July celebration as bursts of blinding light filled the universe. He was aware of hands grasping him, guiding him. Everything spun out of control.

When reality had righted itself, Ira found himself back in bed, atop the crumpled sheets. He started to stir, then felt his fingers brush against something. It was his pistol. He closed his hand around it, then opened his eyes. It took a mighty effort to raise his head.

David Vandemark was sitting in a chair on the far side of the room, his arms folded calmly across his chest. He looked like a solemn cigar-store Indian that someone had spirited into the room while Ira slept.

Ira sat up in bed. "Expected to hear from you again, but not this soon. No firepower tonight?"

The cigar-store Indian spoke: "Bad manners to come asking for someone's help while holding a gun on them."

Ira trained his weapon on David and said, "You won't mind if I cover you with mine while we talk?"

"Not if it makes you feel better. But by the time we finish, you'll realize you could be putting that weapon to better uses."

"Okay, talk. What do you want? Another name run?"

David smiled. "No, it's going to be a lot tougher than that, I'm afraid. I want you to help me break into a top-secret government installation."

"Hey, no sweat. Want to do it now or later?"

"Later. I've got a story to tell you first."

"Mind if I put my pants on before you begin?"

"Be my guest."

∞∞∞

"You know what I've been doing for the last seven years, so you know the type of scum I've dealt with. They all pale beside the nest of rats I've uncovered this time."

"Camden?" Ira asked.

"And eight others." David recited the list of names that Dr. Shelley had given him. Ira recognized the two at the end.

"That last man's a U.S. senator!" Ira said in a hushed whisper. "He's on one of the armed forces subcommittees. And the guy before that used to work at the White House." Ira's dream was coming back to haunt him.

"Yeah, he used to be Project Jack's administration liaison. Now he's a fund-raiser for the project."

"You're not trying to tell me Bush had something to do with it?"

"No, I doubt it. From what I've discovered, Ollie North might not have been the only loose cannon during the Reagan-Bush years. I think a lot of people working in

Washington had their own private agendas. They just got more carried away with this one."

Ira shifted uncomfortably in his seat as he considered the implications of what David Vandemark had said. "Before we go any further down that avenue of speculation, you better fill me in on exactly what Project Jack is and how it's connected to the Latino Family Murders."

"Project Jack and the Latino Family Murders are one and the same."

David proceeded to lay out everything he had learned, again failing to mention that he'd used telepathic powers to gain this knowledge, implying instead that he had come by most of it through bribery and threats. David ended his tale by pulling out a mini tape recorder from his coat pocket and playing back the late Dr. Herbert Shelley's confession. He flipped the recorder off before the room could fill with the sound of David's bullet blowing the good doctor's brains out.

Looking into Ira's mind, David was pleased to learn that the FBI agent had concluded that the business at the beginning of the tape was David prompting the interviewee with pieces of information Vandemark already knew. He also saw that the tape had achieved his desired goal: Ira's gun lay on the night table, forgotten.

Ira's expression was somewhere between shock and bewilderment. It wasn't that he thought David was lying. In fact, Vandemark's track record, together with the calm and earnest manner in which he had laid out his case, had made Agent Levitt a believer. He'd been halfway there before David opened his mouth. Ira wasn't naive enough to believe he lived in the land of the brave, the free, and the morally spotless. His time with the Bureau had taught him that few people who sought power did so for altruistic reasons. Charles Camden wasn't the first man to misuse his authority and try to excuse his actions by invoking national security or political expediency. Vandemark's story had the dull ring of truth to it.

But there was too much of it to swallow at one sitting. The sheer brazenness and the enormity of the crime were staggering. Ira's circuits were overloading.

Ira pulled himself together enough to ask, "What did you do with Shelley?"

"Killed him. Couldn't have him running back to Camden and spilling the beans."

Ira stared long and hard at his companion. He couldn't believe he was calmly sitting with a man who had just confessed to murder and that he—Ira Levitt, FBI agent—wasn't going to do anything about it. As a matter of fact, he was actually contemplating aiding this man in committing further felonies. This was nuts!

But then so was a world that could allow something like Project Jack to exist.

It had to be exposed, regardless of the cost.

And the cost would be high. This would surely ruin what was left of his career with the Bureau. So long, pension. He could say good-bye to his friends on the job and many off the job as well. They wouldn't understand, couldn't understand, even after all the facts came out. Old drinking buddies would call him a whistle-blower, a traitor, and worse. Second thoughts began to rear their ugly heads. Was he ready for these consequences? Was he strong enough to see this through? Was it worth the price he would have to pay?

"Why'd you come to me for help?" Ira asked after a time.

David smiled. "Because you're an honest man, Levitt. That probably sounds pretty funny coming from me. But the truth is, I'm a much better judge of character than anyone would believe, and I can tell that right and wrong mean something to you. If we can get our hands on evidence that Project Jack exists, you won't allow it to be buried under a mountain of governmental crap. You'll do something with it."

"Things that you can't do?"

"Evidence from a wanted murderer wouldn't hold up well in anyone's eyes. But if that same proof came from a G-man it would be hard to ignore."

Ira silently cursed David Vandemark. The man was right. Ira was trapped. He had to help Vandemark, this man he'd been hunting for seven years. There was no way out. Ira Levitt was a prisoner of his own conscience. The course of action he was about to embark on ran contrary to all his training and professional judgment. But a part of him held a higher allegiance to doing the right thing than his professional self held to the Bureau and the government. What Camden and his pals were doing was wrong in every sense of the word. The public had to know the truth. The lid had to be blown off Project Jack.

In a hushed, almost conspiratorial voice, Ira said, "So what do we do next?"

David grinned. "Tomorrow you scour New York City for a wet suit that you can get your overweight self into. Leave the rest to me."

PART THREE

Styx

The world itself is but a large prison, out of which some are daily led to execution.

—Sir Walter Raleigh

41

David sat on a West Side pier, his legs dangling over the edge. He was more than ten blocks north of Camden's installation—well out of range of any video spy cameras, he hoped. He munched hungrily on a deli sandwich, resting as he ate. He'd expended a great deal of energy today and was hoping some food would recharge the old batteries. The sun was setting over the buildings on the Jersey side of the river. It wouldn't be long before he'd be going to work. The night shift.

The end product of his day's labors floated below him, tied to the pier. No one would guess its real purpose. He'd done a much better camouflage job on it than Camden's people had done with their spy cameras.

David leaned back against a piling and closed his eyes. As tired as he was, he didn't worry about falling asleep. Anticipation of tonight's festivities kept a steady, comfortable level of adrenaline coursing through his veins—not enough to make him jittery but enough to give him a nice edge.

Or was he kidding himself?

David weighed that possibility carefully. Everything

about this case was off-kilter. David anticipated serious problems. This wasn't some group of half-baked loonies. These fully baked ones had friends in high places. Hell, they might be in high places themselves. In any case it looked as if that ultimate white-hatted hero, the U.S. government, might be on the wrong side this time. That was problem number one.

Problem number two was the fact that his quarry was aware of him. How aware? David wasn't sure. Did Camden know who he was? Now, that was the $64,000 question. This was the first time David had ever had a target turn on him before he was ready to strike. He didn't like the feeling one bit. His fingers touched his raw neck. Those goons shouldn't have been able to get that close to him. He'd screwed up. That was problem number three.

David knew he wasn't firing on all cylinders. His performance so far on this case had been well below par. He'd allowed himself to be roughed up, almost captured by the law, and then damn near killed. The few chuckles he'd managed along the way hardly made up for the embarrassment he felt at having been handled like some rank amateur. On this job you could be having the greatest day of your life and still kiss your ass good-bye thanks to some tiny oversight.

David knew what was causing the problem: Angela. She'd quietly insinuated herself into his life, and her unexpected presence made all the difference. She was drawing him back into a world where all the norms applied. And that was dulling his edge. The all-important compulsion wasn't there anymore. And that fact could very well get him killed. But he wouldn't have had it any other way.

Things were moving so quickly. He'd met her only a few

short days ago. But David knew that he was in love with Angela Quinoñes. And he was sure she felt the same way. Was it kismet? Destiny? Whatever it was, he and Angela were meant to be together. And somehow they would be. How they would accomplish this minor miracle was another matter, one that would need to be worked out later. After he'd concluded this affair with the Slasher, he would be free to plight his troth. What a romantic sap you are, Vandemark. Anyone ever mention that to you?

❧ A car pulled up to the far end of the pier and parked. Ira was right on time. Dark blue sedan straight off the assembly line, those tiny standard hubcaps, no frills, no extras. No one but a government car pool would own such a vehicle. A moment later Ira stepped out of the car and ambled toward him, carrying a knapsack under his arm.

David had stayed in Ira's hotel room until very late last night, going over the plan. It had taken some serious arm-twisting to make the FBI agent agree that raiding the installation was necessary. Levitt had wanted to find a way to work things out legally. But eventually he'd had to admit that any proof would be shredded or burned before they could reach it through regular channels. It was time to play the covert-action game, to step outside the law. Time to enter David Vandemark's area of expertise. If they didn't, more innocents would die.

Once they got started on the actual planning, Ira had contributed some excellent ideas. He spotted the holes in David's plan and filled them with professional suggestions. David suspected that years of going by the book had enhanced a latent talent for burglary. He wondered how many times Levitt had stewed over a case, knowing he could crack it in record time if only he wasn't constrained by the laws concerning illegal search and seizure. This case was giving Ira a chance to purge years' worth of frustration.

When he and Ira had finished their strategy session, David found a pay phone outside the FBI agent's hotel and called Angela. He could hear the disappointment and fear in her voice when he informed her he wouldn't be coming home tonight. David assured her that nothing dangerous was going on. He had to talk to a possible witness up in Yonkers. It would be easier if he found a hotel room tonight. He would see Angela late tomorrow night. There was absolutely nothing for her to worry about. David almost fooled himself into believing she bought his story.

Lying to Angela felt lousy, but he would square it with her later. For now he grabbed a cab over to Angela's block. There were few people on the street at this time of night. David gave each of them a perfunctory telepathic scan before heading for the garage. They came up clean. Camden had called off his dogs once they'd located, photographed, and mapped Angela's apartment. So David got the impression that this neighborhood was a safe haven.

David stopped at the garage teller's window and paid for another two days' parking. Saying he wanted to get a few things out of the van, he wandered up to the top level of the garage and climbed into his portable private refuge. The attendant on duty would think he'd missed Vandemark's leaving while busy doing something else.

David had rolled out a sleeping bag and crawled into it. He regretted his decision to spend the night here rather than in the comfort of Angela's warm bed, but he was positive it was the right thing to do. Tomorrow would be filled with work, danger, and possibly death. He'd have to be at his peak. This move would spare him the hassle of having to explain his bandaged neck. More important, he wasn't sure he'd be able to conceal other unpleasant facts from Angela face to face. Trying to con her over the phone had been tough enough.

Sooner or later he would have to come clean and let her know what he really did for a living—if that's what you could call it.

The only hope for them was if David told her everything. But what would happen then? He doubted even a woman as strong as Angela could handle having her husband taking off for months at a time on these little jobs. It wasn't exactly like marrying a traveling salesman. Taking her along on these forays was out of the question. Sometime in the not-too-distant future he would have to make a choice between his calling and his woman, and he knew what his decision would be.

In the morning he was awakened by attendants parking the cars of early-morning commuters. Thinking about what lay ahead of him that day, he rolled over and caught another two hours of sleep. There was no telling when he'd get the opportunity again. This day could easily become a forty-eight-hour marathon.

When he did get up, he dressed in work clothes, ready to take on the grimy job ahead. His backpack was filled with weapons, tools, and miscellaneous items.

He ate a hearty brunch at a local greasy spoon neighborhood coffee shop while he read the papers. They didn't report anything new about the Slasher, but there was an item about a group of local politicians who were gathering petitions calling for the mayor's resignation. The editorial page carried a scathing piece on how badly the city government was handling the Latino Family Murders. Many of the facts in the piece were incorrect, but David knew this wouldn't matter to the people who wanted to oust the mayor. New York was a city in the grip of fear, and people needed a scapegoat, someone to vent their frustration on. It looked as if the mayor had been chosen as the fall guy.

After brunch he made a quick stop at a sporting-goods outlet, where he bought a wet suit.

The rest of the morning was spent gathering the materials he needed to build a boat. He then worked most of the afternoon on his vessel, but the results were well worth the effort. The craft was moored to the pier by a length of baling wire. It bobbed in the choppy waters of the Hudson River.

David had used scrap wood and cardboard from nearby Dumpsters. From an abandoned warehouse he'd procured an empty wooden packing crate, which had become the centerpiece of his creation. He'd stuffed a discarded fifty-gallon fuel drum into the crate for buoyancy. He had created a rickety stern and bow from scrap wood and secured it in place with nails and wire. The craft sat in the water, looking like a collection of refuse that had snarled itself into a shape only a modern abstract sculptor could appreciate. But David hadn't been striving for aesthetic integrity. His creation was a triumph of function over form.

❧❧❧

As David watched Ira Levitt lumber down the pier, he wondered what the FBI agent would think of his craft. Not much, he supposed, until its wondrous workings were explained to him. But as Ira neared, David noticed something different about the man. It took him a second or two to pinpoint the change. The burly agent dropped his bundle onto the dock with an exaggerated thunk and waited for David's comment.

"Agent Levitt, you look positively half dressed without your cast."

Ira smiled as he flexed his plasterless hand. "Yeah, it feels great to be rid of it."

"How's the arm?"

"Not as strong as it should be, but it'll do. The cast was scheduled to come off next week anyhow. Got a jeweler's saw and did the deed myself. I wouldn't have been able to get into the wet suit otherwise."

Ira sat down on the pier and looked toward the setting sun. "How long do you suppose we have to wait before going in?"

"Let's give ourselves an hour after the sun sets."

"Sounds good to me." Ira pulled a white paper bag out of his knapsack. "Brought along a couple of sandwiches. Want one?"

"No thanks. I already ate dinner."

Ira dug in as both men settled back to watch the sun dip behind the New Jersey skyline. Neither spoke for a while. Both wondered briefly whether they'd be around tomorrow when the sun set again, but they immediately dispensed with such thoughts. Tonight's work would be hard enough without carrying along a lot of what-ifs.

As the last rays of sunlight disappeared, Ira said, "After we're finished with Camden, what do you plan to do?"

David returned Ira's gaze without answering.

"You realize our truce will end when we expose Camden's scam. After that it's back to the old hunter-and-hunted relationship, David. Is that how you want it?"

Vandemark stared out at the river. "No. As a matter of fact, I'm considering giving up the life after we're done here."

Ira couldn't hide his surprise. He felt his jaw go slack. Was their seven-year game of hide-and-seek going to conclude so anticlimactically? Ira would have been more than pleased if things worked out that way, but he had never even entertained the possibility. It was inconceivable. Almost.

"What brought this on?" Ira asked hesitantly.

"I met a woman."

"She must be something."

"She is. I guess I'm planning to spend the rest of my life with her."

"Well, I'll do everything I can to help out, David. I'll be a character witness at your trial, and I'll make it go as easy as I can for you."

"Thanks, Ira. But I see no reason to go through the hassle of a trial at taxpayers' expense. I don't think anyone would want me to go that route."

Again Ira was dumbstruck. When he found his voice he said, "How you figure that? There're twenty counts of murder pending against you, not counting Herbert Shelley."

"Twenty counts of murdering serial killers, Ira. What judge or jury would want to slap a life sentence on me for getting rid of that trash?"

"How about those two cops you shot in Nevada and my broken arm?"

"Extenuating circumstances. Besides, what proof do you have that I did that?"

Ira realized, with some irritation, that the answer to that question was "None." The policemen had been shot with Ira's gun, which had never been recovered, and he himself had never gotten a good look at David that night.

David winked at Ira, smiling broadly. "Buck up, old pal. It isn't as bad as all that. Besides, I imagine both those cops are back on their feet by now, your arm's working fine, and everyone has learned to be more careful. Where's the harm? I think that was a small price to pay for the cleanup job I did."

"But—but the law . . ." Ira stammered.

"Fuck the law!" snapped David. "Your law didn't catch those killers. *I* did. They're not murdering anyone anymore. I'll take justice over the law any day. And I'm willing to bet the twelve men and women on a jury would see it my way."

"Yeah, a good lawyer would most likely get you off with an insanity plea. The court would probably insist you spend some time under psychiatric care."

"That'll never happen. And if it did, those psychiatrists would certify me cured in two months' time," David said with confidence.

Before Ira could follow this train of thought, David leaped to his feet and pointed over the edge of the pier. "I want you to inspect my handiwork before it gets too dark for you to appreciate it."

Ira looked at the pile of debris floating in the water. "What the hell is that?"

"That's the submarine I promised you. Ahoy, mate!"

42

Last night Camden had gone to bed confident the entire Vandemark matter would be settled by the following evening. It would be a permanent solution to the problems that troubled young man was wreaking on Camden's plans and timetable.

But now Camden didn't feel quite so certain. This day had been a royal pain in the ass. Every time he turned around a new crisis arose.

When Shelley didn't show up for work, Camden sent a couple of his men to the doctor's apartment, where they questioned Herbert's housekeeper. They learned that Dr. Shelley's bed hadn't been slept in the night before and the usual breakfast dishes weren't sitting in the sink, awaiting her arrival. Camden had to conclude that Vandemark had gotten to Herbert Shelley sometime last night.

That left some questions hanging in the ether unanswered. For instance, how had Vandemark found out where Shelley lived? And where had he taken the doctor? How much had Herbert told Vandemark? Camden had no illusions how well Herbert Shelley would hold up under interrogation. A little pain and that sniveling intellectual weakling would spill his guts. Camden cursed himself for not having sent a couple of bodyguards over to Shelley's last night. But how was he to have known that Vandemark had such good intelligence on Camden's outfit? Around noon it dawned on Camden that some traitor in his organization had to be leaking info to Vandemark. But there was no time to find out who this Benedict Arnold was right now. Vandemark had to be dealt with first. Then the turncoat could be ferreted out.

Camden had his police contacts put APBs out on Vandemark and Shelley. David Vandemark was to be considered armed and dangerous. Herbert Shelley was probably his captive. If at all possible, no harm was to come to this second man. The police officials asked no questions.

But the wheels of the NYPD moved slowly, and Camden didn't learn of Herbert Shelley's death until nearly three o'clock. A man walking his Saint Bernard in Central Park had discovered Shelley's body early that morning.

Camden decided that Vandemark would not have killed Shelley until he had everything he needed from the scientist. This meant that he was more dangerous than ever. But what could Vandemark, a wanted criminal, do with the information he had? He couldn't take it to the police. Newspapers presented the same problem, as no one would run a story blowing the whistle on a federal agency when their only source was a psychotic killer. Vandemark could use his newly gained knowledge only if he stayed in character. This meant that the vigilante would be coming after him. Camden could handle that.

The security force at the installation was doubled.

Once the sun had set, it was tripled. An army of paid gunmen would keep David Vandemark at bay.

Surveillance on the Quiñones apartment had been set in place around noon. There had been nothing to report from that front since earlier this evening, when Angela Quiñones had returned home from work. She had left again almost immediately. An operative followed her to a neighborhood grocery store, where she picked up what was probably dinner for two. She then returned to the apartment. But the operatives had no idea what was going on inside the apartment or who was there. The drapes had been drawn throughout the day.

Which meant David Vandemark might or might not be there.

A high-tech directional spy microphone had been hurried over to the stakeout, but so far its operators had picked up only classical music from the stereo. Was Vandemark there? Just because they hadn't heard any conversation didn't mean that Angela Quiñones was alone. The reports Camden had read regarding yesterday's attempt on Vandemark's life stated that he hadn't escaped the encounter unscathed. Vandemark could be laid up in that apartment, licking his wounds, perhaps sleeping.

Charles Camden sat at his desk, brooding over this dilemma. If Vandemark was in that apartment, Camden could send in the hit team and everything would be taken care of. Vandemark and the girl would be eliminated and all problems solved. A nice tidy package. But if Vandemark was out, killing the girl would warn him off. He would go underground. It might take years to find him again, and there was no telling what damage he could cause in the interim. Project Jack would have to be scrubbed.

Camden decided that doing nothing was the greater of these two evils. The hit team would have to go in. If that psycho wasn't there, they could shove the Quiñones woman's body into a closet and wait for Vandemark's return. Maybe Camden would get lucky and Vandemark would show up at the installation again. He could be dealt with here as easily as at the apartment.

Either way, David Vandemark would be a dead man by sunrise and Camden could once again rest easy. Then Project Jack would continue without further delay. Everything would work out. The cards were stacked in Camden's favor. He couldn't lose.

Charles Camden checked his watch. The time was 8:15 P.M.

43

It was eight-fifteen and David had not returned. Angela walked to the window and searched the street below through the gap in the drapes. Still no sign of him, just as there had been no sign of him two minutes ago. Angela promised herself this would be her last trip to the window.

There was nothing to worry about, she told herself. David had said he would be home late. Angela kicked herself for not having pinned him down to a more specific time of arrival. But she couldn't have done that. She and David didn't know each other well enough for her to be acting like a wife.

Like a wife? Yes, that was definitely where this was heading. She'd never been here before, but she recognized the terrain. She and David were headed for happily ever after. She could feel it in her blood, see it in his eyes. But was that what she wanted?

Angela looked at her lonely apartment, with the drapes shut, closeted off from the rest of the world. Sharing her life with David would mean many moments like this, sitting alone, wondering if he'd make it home alive. This had to be how the wives of policemen felt. In time she would find things to fill the void created by his absence. She would keep herself busy while he was gone and wouldn't think about the dangers. Then he'd return and lie about how everything had gone smoothly. They would share some wonderful times together. But life would be a vicious cycle of glorious reunions followed by anxious separations and waiting, long days of waiting and fretting. Angela wondered if she was strong enough to lead such a life.

She saw David's smiling face in her mind's eye, and all her soul-searching seemed a waste of time. What choice did she have? How could she live without him?

● Angela stepped into the kitchen once more to make certain everything was set for dinner when David returned. Yes, the fish needed only fifteen minutes in the oven, the vegetables ten minutes on the stovetop, and their banquet would be ready. So she poured herself a glass of wine and returned to the living room.

As she sipped at her drink, her eye was caught by the photo of Jeffrey Parker, her former fiancé. Instead of simply passing by it, as she so often had, she picked it up. It wasn't easy to admit, but Jeffrey's departure had been a lucky break for her. The marriage never would have worked out. Parker was a wild and glorious child. He had swept Angela off her feet with his cocaine-stoked devil-may-care style. Every minute spent with Jeffrey had been filled with excitement. This was part of her attraction to David as well. It was a different kind of excitement, but the thrill was there.

Jeffrey Parker had shown his irresponsible streak early in the courtship. He was always late. He forgot Angela's twenty-sixth birthday, but he bought her a wonderful present the next day. They'd been going together for two years when that happened. And then there were those little things she asked him to do that never got done. But if, God forbid, she failed to do his laundry on time or some other little task he'd somehow sweet talked her into, he made her feel as if she'd let him down, as if he saw her failure to serve him promptly as some kind of personal affront.

Angela knew she should have left him, but he was so damn charming when things were going right. When he wasn't being an ass, Jeffrey would whisk her away to a world of champagne and bright lights. He'd shown her parts of New York she never knew existed. They had flown to the Caribbean one weekend. Another favorite memory was of Jeffrey driving her down to South Ferry at three in the morning to see how beautiful the Statue of Liberty looked with the moon glowing directly above it.

But Jeffrey had revealed his true colors too often. Angela understood that he couldn't help himself. He'd spent a lifetime being pampered by his well-to-do parents, and he expected the same treatment from her. A share in the exuberant chaos that was Jeffrey Parker was to be her sole reward.

Angela finally decided she'd had enough. She was waiting for the right moment to break it off. She'd decided to let Jeffrey down easy. She didn't hate the guy; she just wanted him out of her life. That was when fate intervened.

The police had caught Jeffrey in his office men's room with his precious little vial of coke clutched in one hand, a spoon in the other, and three grams of incriminating evidence in his briefcase. Without warning, Jeffrey was out of her life. It.was the first time he'd ever done anything for her, without having to be asked at least half a dozen times.

She couldn't think of Jeffrey without the word *irrespon-sible* popping into her head. It had been an uncomfortably narrow escape.

But with David, Angela felt that life would be differ-ent. Sure, there'd be the anxious hours of waiting. But she knew in her heart that if she ever needed him for any-thing he would be there for her.

David might even give up his line of work if she asked him nicely, but that wasn't Angela's style. She wasn't into re-creating her men. Smoothing out the rough edges was okay, but a full-blown makeover was out of the question. She would take them as she found them or not at all.

Angela got up from her chair to walk to the window, then remembered her promise and went over to the book-shelf instead. She picked up a thick novel she'd been chipping away at. "Read!" she commanded herself. "It'll take your mind off the time."

She struggled through two pages of the story, didn't re-call anything she'd read, and gave up, returning the book to its place on the shelf. Maybe there was something on the tube. She switched on the television and flipped through the dozens of channels New York's cable system offered up for her amusement, settling for some old car-toons on the Disney Channel. The antics of Donald, Goofy, and Mickey would keep her amused without de-manding anything of her. They don't make cartoons like this anymore, she thought.

The hands on the clock continued to crawl. At nine o'clock the cartoons ended and Angela flipped to a movie on another channel. Somehow she would make it through this night.

44

Getting Ira into his wet suit was a two-man job. For a while it looked as if the suit might not be large enough. Ira kept complaining loudly, "The salesman assured me it'd be big enough! Said it was the largest size they had in stock." After much huffing and puffing, they got the outfit zipped. Ira looked like a large blue whale with legs. David's suit was jet black. Both would disappear nicely beneath the Hudson's murky waters.

As Ira lowered himself off the pier, he swore he'd lose at least thirty pounds after this affair. A man his size wasn't meant to take on this kind of cloak-and-dagger stuff. David was inclined to agree. If Ira thought this part of the job was tough, wait until they got to the installation. David wondered why he hadn't teamed up with Vida instead. At least she looked physically fit.

But when he'd first looked into Vida Johnson's mind, David knew she'd never go along with an idea as crazy as this one. She was too much of a straight arrow; she wouldn't dream of bending the rules. Vida had too much to lose.

So it was Ira or nothing. Somehow David would make it work.

He showed Ira how to duck beneath the water and come up inside the "submarine," inside the enclosure for his head. This would allow him to breathe without a snorkel while they traveled downriver to Camden's headquarters. From the depths of the ramshackle construction of driftwood, Ira's voice echoed hollowly. "I can't see a fucking thing in here!"

"You don't have to. I'll do the navigating from the bow. My compartment's got a peep hole."

David heard Ira submerge. A moment later Levitt bobbed up to the surface outside the craft, where he got a grip on a piling. "Why do we need this contraption? Can't we just swim to the warehouse?"

"Because I don't know what kind of surveillance equipment Camden's got covering the river. It might be a video camera with a nightscope, or the lens might be infrared. If it's the latter, the water will mask most of our body heat. This submarine will hide the heat signatures of our heads. I know it's crude, but it might work."

"And if it doesn't?"

"How fast can you swim, Ira?"

❧❧❧❧

Earlier in the day, David had prepared two bundles and wrapped them tightly in black plastic. Now he secured them to the submarine below the waterline. He checked his watch: 9:08 P.M. "Time to shove off, Ira. You coming?"

"Sure, why not," said Ira, eyeing the floating scrap heap. "Everybody needs meshugass in their life now and then. But before we go, tell me one thing. This Project Jack, it wouldn't perhaps draw its name from the Ripper in White Castle?"

"Whitechapel."

"Whatever . . ."

Even in this poor light Ira could see David's smile broaden. "*Vo den?*"

"Cute," said Ira. "You know 'what else' in Yiddish. You're full of surprises, aren't you?"

"Chock full." David disappeared beneath the water. A few moments later Ira heard him come up inside the pilot compartment. A voice from inside the not-so-stately craft said, "We'll have no trouble getting downriver from here. The tide doesn't change for another hour."

"What the hell's the tide got to do with anything? This is a river, not an ocean!"

"This, my crotchety friend," said the voice, "is the Hudson River. Most of its length is at sea level. An hour from now the tide will change. When that happens, the Hudson starts running upstream for about fifty miles north. So if we have to run for it anytime after ten o'clock, remember to head upriver. Okay?"

"You shittin' me?"

"No. Get in here. We're shoving off."

Ira clung to his piling, grimly contemplating the submarine's dark hulk. Rivers that ran the wrong way. Breaking into a top-secret government installation with a homicidal maniac. Taking on Charles Camden. He just kept getting in deeper and deeper. So what do you have in mind for an encore? he asked himself.

Ira disappeared into the inky depths of the Hudson and reemerged inside his own private eighteen-inch-square private stateroom aboard the good ship Looney Tunes. "Okay. Let's do it."

A voice from the bow of the vessel answered, "Anchors aweigh! Full speed dead ahead!"

And they were off.

❧❧❧

Chester Pinyon was doing a double shift on the monitors tonight, sixteen hours straight. The first eight hours had been a breeze. Now it seemed an awful long time until midnight, when Jerry Stillson was scheduled to relieve him. Chester had traded his Saturday-afternoon shift with another security guard so he could have the entire weekend off. There was a gallery opening on Long Island he wanted to attend. It'd be a chance to schmooze with the owner and maybe talk him into showing some of Chester's masterpieces.

Chester was at the stage in his career where exposure was critical. The great unwashed masses would never realize the true genius he possessed if he didn't get his paintings out before the public's eye. But that was a frustratingly difficult goal to achieve. Those small-minded gallery owners kept telling him that he wasn't quite ready for a show. Maybe in a year or so, they said. But Chester knew what their game was. He knew the radical quality of his work would make the mediocre dabblings making up the inventories of most galleries pale in comparison. But this turkey out on Long Island might be willing to take a chance on him. Maybe he would prove to be Chester's stepping-stone to fame, fortune, and the good life. Chester wished he could remember the guy's name. Well, someone at the opening would be able to refresh his memory.

On his way back from the coffee machine Chester wondered why it couldn't produce something that tasted vaguely like coffee. Sure, this stuff would keep him awake until midnight, but he didn't want to think about the damage this acidic brew was doing to his insides. One of the gorillas, Pete Braddock, was spelling him at the console. Gorillas—that was what the regular security guards called Mr. Camden's boys. Never to their faces, of course.

Chester didn't like leaving any of the gorillas at the monitors for very long. They had terribly short attention spans. Left too long in front of the multiple screens, they tended to fall asleep. Sensory overload, Chester figured. Too much for their pea-sized brains to handle.

The only thing worse than their falling asleep was when one of these idiot goons decided to adjust the image on a monitor. Hey, why shouldn't they give it a shot? They'd fixed the picture on their own TV sets dozens of times. So what if their Sonys didn't have half the adjustment knobs the monitors had? A TV's a TV, right? The gorillas had been known to screw up the picture so badly it would take Chester several hours to get a clear image again. Now they had specific orders to sit, watch, and not touch anything. But sometimes the temptation was too great.

As he stepped into the monitor room, Chester gave all the screens a quick once-over. His eye locked on the screen showing a view of the Hudson River just north of the installation. "What's that on screen eight?" he asked.

Braddock leaned forward in his seat and stared myopically at the screen. "What you talkin' about? I don't see nothin'!"

Chester stepped over to the console and calmly pushed the appropriate buttons to enhance the image of the mysterious object that was drifting down the Hudson River toward the installation.

"Looks like junk to me," offered Braddock.

Chester continued to watch the screen without responding. "Yes," he said after a few moments. "Just driftwood and scrap."

The Hudson River monitors picked up the oddest things floating up- and downstream. Chester had once spotted a department-store mannequin floating by, which he mistook for a dead body and he'd immediately hit the alarm button. This conscientious act had won him the nickname "Dummy Pinyon" for several weeks afterward.

Chester was glad they'd installed high-powered nightscope lenses on the cameras. They cut through the darkness to produce nearly crystal-clear images on the screens.

Sipping his coffee, Chester wondered if he should enter the driftwood into the log. Normally he wouldn't bother. But tonight wasn't normal. Though everything was quiet, security had been tripled inside the installation. Something was up. Chester had no idea what. But it had to be big to justify all the activity. So he decided to cover his ass. He noted the floating scrap, certain he'd be entering it again when it drifted back upriver an hour from now.

❧❧❧❧

As soon as they were under the section of warehouse that extended out over the river, David popped up from beneath his homemade craft. He whispered for Ira to join him. David grabbed Ira as soon as he broke the surface and signaled him to remain quiet. He retrieved the two packages from underneath the sub and wedged them into diagonal support beams above the waterline. When he finished, he pushed his craft back out into the current and watched it drift away.

❧❧❧❧

In the monitor room, Chester viewed the floating scrap heap's departure on screen number nine.

❧❧❧❧

David left Ira clinging to a piling and began a careful recon of the waters below the warehouse, searching for video cameras. He found none and returned to Ira without having to damage any federal property. Typical government efficiency, he decided. Don't bother to put a surveillance camera at your most vulnerable point: your underbelly.

When David gave him the all clear, Ira clambered up onto a crossbeam, about a foot above the water. There would be nothing for him to do for a while, so he might as well get comfortable. From his perch, he got a better view of his surroundings, but it was too dark underneath the warehouse to make out details. He could just make out the network of support beams that held the installation above the water, but not much else. It looked like an ongoing battle to keep the warehouse from falling into the river. The entire support structure was jury-rigged. Layers of crossbeams were strapped to pilings. Newer diagonal and vertical beams were in evidence. Ira guessed that in a year or two the whole shebang would collapse into the Hudson and float out to sea.

David circled back to the warehouse carrying the two bundles. He came to a stop when he heard a deep-throated rumble above him: the installation's generator. Herbert Shelley had said that Camden didn't trust New York's iffy electrical power, so one of his first official acts had been to install a generator. It kept a meter reader from poking his nose where it didn't belong.

Dr. Shelley had provided a wealth of useful information, bless his black soul.

David shimmied up a piling to an overhead crossbeam. The vertical timber was about four feet from the under-flooring of the warehouse. From the larger of the two bundles David produced some tools and laid them carefully on the crossbeam. He glanced at Ira. The FBI agent had his back against a piling and appeared to have settled in for the night. David hoped Ira wouldn't fall asleep. He looked way too comfortable.

There wasn't time to worry about that now. Squatting, David picked up a monstrous old-fashioned hand-cranked drill and inspected it. The inch-and-a-half-diameter bit was secure in its ten-inch shaft. He raised the tool above his head and began drilling into the warehouse flooring, cutting easily through the dry, rotted boards.

A few minutes later the bit hit the next level of flooring, which was made of newer, more solid wood. This was much slower, harder going. David set up a steady rhythm to pace himself. There was no time for a lot of starts and stops. He worked without fear of discovery. The generator, above and a little to the right of him, would mask the noise.

Ten minutes later David felt the drill break through. He marked the bit with chalk and twisted it free—seven inches of flooring above him.

The thin skillsaw fit snugly into the drill hole. It took David an hour to make a crosscut of about eighteen inches. Then he glanced at Ira, still resting comfortably on his crossbeam. David took another fifteen minutes to add four more inches to the width of his handiwork.

He found he could pull away the first layer of flooring by hand. It crumbled into dusty splinters as he tore it loose. But the boards above were so solid that he couldn't even pry them loose with a tire iron. He would have to drill another hole and make another crosscut. That was okay, since David had allowed for this eventuality in his timetable. He looked at his watch: 10:26. At this rate the breaking and entering wouldn't yield results until after midnight, but that was all for the best. The later he and Ira invaded Camden's sanctuary, the more lulled into false security his sentries would be.

I'll be damned! thought David, glancing at Ira. The son of a bitch was asleep!

❧❧❧❧❧

Charles Camden faced the three men on the other side of his desk. McGuire and Hanson were relaxed, not listening to the gibberish the third man was spouting. Camden was only half listening himself. Camden wasn't a scientist and had little tolerance for the indecipherable jargon scientists loved. It was enough that Dr. James Hoover, the late Dr. Shelley's assistant, felt confident his charge was ready for this evening's festivities.

Camden would have felt more secure if Shelley were alive to supervise the outing. But Hoover had been with the project from the beginning, and Dr. Shelley had proclaimed his assistant capable of handling the subtle intricacies of Project Jack. Besides, Camden had no choice. His faith was in this second stringer now. The leader of the A-team was dead.

When Hoover finished his report, Camden glanced at McGuire and Hanson and said, "You know what to do?"

"Wait until all lights in the building are extinguished, then take Baby in. Back him up, let him take them out if he can. If Vandemark's not there, wait for him and finish the job when he arrives."

"You've got it. Good luck."

Both men left with Dr. Hoover in tow. No sooner had the door closed behind them than Camden's intercom buzzed. He flipped the switch. "Yes?"

"Stevens in personnel, sir. We've got a problem. Jerry Stillson, the monitor on tonight's graveyard shift, called in sick a little while ago. Apparently he caught that bug that's going around."

"Get to the point, Stevens."

"Yes, sir. I've been calling around for a replacement, but I can't find anyone at home."

"Then have the man currently on duty stay another shift."

"That's Pinyon, sir. He's been on for nearly sixteen hours already. Chester's pretty beat."

"Have someone bring him some amphetamines from the medical station. I need a trained man on those monitors tonight. Have one of the security men stay with him to make sure he doesn't nod off. Anything else?"

"No, sir. Just wanted to check with you before—"

Camden flipped off the intercom. He looked up at the Gainsborough on the wall. Nothing to do now but wait.

❧❧❧

Ira Levitt wasn't asleep. Years of stakeouts had taught him how to relax without dozing off. Waiting was what cops of all stripes did best. Sure, the crossbeam was hard and uncomfortable, but he'd had worse places in which to wait. On this stakeout at least he had a floor show to keep him entertained.

Watching David Vandemark tear away at that floor was a real treat. The man was attacking the job as if his life depended on it. And Ira supposed that it did. David had told him of the botched attack by Camden's men. That meant Camden had the scent and was after him. With someone like Charles Camden after you, there were only two ways to handle the situation. One: flee to Tibet, find a deep hole to crawl into, and pull the earth over you. Or two: get Camden before he got you. Vandemark had opted for the latter.

Ira considered offering to help Vandemark but decided against it. Too close quarters for more than one person to be working on that beam. And that timber looked too narrow for him to comfortably take David's place. Ira knew his limitations. Besides, he was along as an unofficial observer and backup. Let the younger man do the heavy work. Ira was going to save his strength for later on, when things got hairy.

David was ripping out some of the inner boards now. It wouldn't be long. Ira's watch showed it was a little past midnight.

❧❧❧❧❧❧

Angela couldn't stave off her hunger any longer with wine. It wouldn't do to be potted when David got back. So around eleven o'clock she cooked her half of the dinner and ate it. But it was a dismal meal, reminding her of the solitary dinners she'd endured over the recent months. That was going to change soon.

After doing the dishes, Angela considered going to bed. It might be nice to have David find her warm, cozy, and sleepy, safe within the silken confines of their love nest.

But Angela was too wired to sleep. If she stayed up, she could find something to keep her mind occupied. A half dozen movies came on the tube at 11:30. Maybe one of them would be a comedy.

Absentmindedly, she wandered to the window. Still no sign of David. In fact, the only activity on the street below was a van pulling up to the curb and two men climbing out. Angela closed the curtain and turned back to the anesthetizing solace of the boob tube.

꘎꘎꘎

The last board ripped away with a crack like a gunshot, showering David with dust and splinters. He stared up at the gaping hole, wondering what lay beyond it. Would his long hours of work reward him with a bullet between the eyes when at last he stuck his head up through that portal? There was no telling if anyone was in the room above. The noisy generator would have obscured the sounds of a person entering as easily as it had masked Vandemark's demolition work.

David signaled Ira to bring over the second plastic-wrapped bundle. While he waited, he dropped his tools into the river's black water, keeping only the tire iron, in case any locked doors had to be coaxed open.

Ira handed up the package. David ripped away its protective covering to reveal a small backpack. From it he pulled two Taurus PT 92s individually wrapped in plastic and two shoulder holsters. Another packet contained two silencers and four additional mags of 9 mm bullets, fifteen to a magazine. He laid all this at the far end of the beam and went over to give Ira a hand up.

Both men slipped into the shoulder harnesses, screwed on the silencers, and holstered the pistols. The holsters were snap-opens with the bottoms cut off to accommodate silencers. The extra ammo hung in pouches from the right shoulder of each harness. David slipped the tire iron into the backpack and put it on.

Nothing left to do except get on with it.

David crawled under his newly created entrance to Charles Camden's domain and stared up into the darkened room above. It didn't look very inviting. He unholstered his gun and gave Ira a look. The FBI agent gave him a thumbs-up, but its meaning was lost on David. Did that upraised thumb indicate that Ira was ready to go? Was it an expression of his confidence in David? Or was Levitt just telling him to get his ass moving? He'd ask Ira later. If there was a "later."

David's psychic powers didn't register anyone in the room above. But he wasn't sure he could trust his special sense so close to that bloody generator. He'd found in the past that he sometimes had trouble reading people when they were around anything involving high-voltage electricity. Someday he'd have a scientist explain it to him. But at the moment there was only one surefire way to find out if anyone was up there.

David poked his head up through the hole in the floor.

Nothing happened. No one shot, clubbed, or grabbed him. But the room was so dark he couldn't be sure whether anyone was there to ambush him. Luckily they would have no way of knowing he was there unless they had night-vision scopes. His continuing existence over the next few seconds assured David they didn't. But they would know he was there the moment he started to crawl into the room. He could see it now. The lights would go on and there he'd be, flat on his face, trying to pull himself out of the hole.

There was no turning back. So David laid his gun on the floorboards and climbed through the hole. Once inside, he picked up his piece and began to feel his way blindly around the room, heading away from the sound of the generator. He reached a wall and made his way along it until he discovered a door. Groping around, he located the light switch and flipped it. The room was filled with a blinding brightness.

He found himself alone in a basic industrial-strength utility room. Big generator cranking away in the center of the space. Oversized furnace to his left. Giant water-heating system to his right. A hole in the floor in front of the generator.

Ira's head popped up out of that hole and slowly surveyed his surroundings. He turned to David. Then in a perfect Bugs Bunny voice, the burly FBI agent said, "Ehhhhhhhhhhhhhh . . . this don't look like Pismo Beach to me, Doc."

45

David hurried over to help his chunky confederate into the room. He grunted and strained as the overweight FBI agent struggled to his feet. That much accomplished, David slapped Ira on the back and said, "Now you're getting into the swing of things, Ira. I like your attitude."

"What the hell? We're taking on one of Washington's biggest powerhouses, jeopardizing both our lives and my career. If you can't have a little fun along the way, why bother?"

"My sentiments exactly. Better get out your hardware. It's time to go exploring."

David's good humor was due to a renewed confidence in his powers. Ira's thoughts were coming through loud and clear. There didn't seem to be any interference from the generator. David went to the door, gently probed for unwanted presences outside it and, finding none, turned the knob to see if it was locked. It wasn't. For Ira's benefit, he stuck his head out to confirm what his more exotic sense had already told him.

It was an empty hallway, one that could've belonged in any government building. "Nondescript" was the operative word here. The bare walls were painted a pea green paint with a touch of gray in it. The hallway had absolutely no character. David stepped back into the utility room and closed the door.

They would have to wait ten minutes or so to let Ira dry off. Puddles of water all over the halls would be like Day-Glo footprints with accompanying signs saying "They went that way!"

As they waited, David reviewed the plan aloud. "Shelley's office is one flight up and down the hall to our left—room 10B. Everything we need is in his file cabinet. We keep our traps shut until we reach the office. Even then keep it down to a whisper. No one's got any reason to come back to this end of the installation at night, but why take chances."

Ira looked silently at David for a few beats, then said, "No killing unless it's absolutely necessary. Understand?"

"Sure, whatever you say."

"I mean it, David. Camden has to be stopped, but I'm not about to take part in a wholesale massacre of what might be innocent technicians."

"I don't slaughter innocents," said David.

"Not even by mistake?"

"I don't make mistakes about life and death."

❧❧❧

They didn't run into any trouble as they made their way down the hall. But as they climbed the stairs David suddenly stiffened. The guy must have some very acute hearing. Probably picks up dog whistles, thought Ira as David hurried him back down the stairs and into the utility room. On the way, Ira heard two voices approaching from the staircase.

The two trespassers stood frozen, listening to the voices pass by the door of the utility room and fade into the distance. Ira grabbed David by the arm and said, "Thought no one would be coming back to this end of the installation. Who were those guys?"

"Camden's expecting us. He's got security patrolling the hallways. Let's move before the next shift comes through."

They sprinted to the stairs and up a flight. Room 10B was at the end of another barren, government-issue corridor. David was surprised to find it unlocked, and he was immensely grateful for the slipshod procedures Camden's security forces employed. They were so sure their surveillance system would keep unwanted visitors out that few interior security measures had been taken.

Dr. Shelley's file cabinet was locked, but it wasn't constructed well enough to keep out a determined man with a tire iron. A lab coat jammed between the bottom of the solid oak door and the floor kept the office lights and their unauthorized presence a secret. Ira and David dumped the file cabinet's contents onto the late doctor's desk and began rifling through them. "We can't take it all," David said. "Have to sort through and pick out the meat. Leave most of the technical crap behind. What we want is proof of Project Jack's existence and intent and anything with Charles Camden's name on it."

"No problem. Looks like he signed or initialed every scrap of paper."

"Well, look what I've got here," whispered David.

"What is it?"

"Dr. Herbert Shelley's thesis, the paper that got this whole ugly mess rolling. You could call it the Fear Paper." Leafing through the thesis, David said, "It's about public hysteria—a very well thought out essay on the psychological effects and sociological ramifications that the Jack the Ripper murders had on the population of 1888 London.

"The Ripper was the first well-publicized killer of his kind. Until then only a few psychosexual murders had occurred in rural areas on the Continent, and they were pretty well hushed up. It says here that Jack was different. He struck in the very heart of a major metropolis, leaving his victims scattered all over the Whitechapel district. The panic he created, fanned by the press, nearly toppled the government."

"How so? I mean, I never heard anything about Jack the Ripper being a revolutionary."

David was skimming furiously. "He wasn't . . . but he created a situation that London's leading revolutionaries used to their advantage. Karl Marx had died five years earlier, but many in London's lower classes were already embracing his ideas with a religious fervor. Remember, London was the birthplace of communism. It was a sociological powder keg at the time. The fact that Jack could strike throughout the city with impunity terrified and inflamed the people. Millions of have-nots were crowded into the city's filthy slums. When they realized the people in power couldn't protect them, they went crazy. There were riots."

David looked up from the paper. "All this sounding a bit familiar?"

"Yeah, too familiar."

"Shelley ends his paper by saying this same mass hysteria could be created within a modern society if the conditions were right."

"Like in New York City?" replied Ira. "Rich and homeless side by side. I don't get it. What's the payoff here? Camden's goal can't be the impeachment of this burg's mayor."

"No, this is just a run-through, an experiment." David was reading again. "Camden's testing Shelley's ideas on expendable people to see if it works before he moves on to his true target population. There ought to be proof of this somewhere in these papers. Keep looking."

There was technical data on drug dosages and conditioning. David salvaged the most important of this material and tossed the rest on the floor. A neat stack of vital documentation was piling up on one corner of the desk.

"Got it! I've found our boy's stats! This is the Slasher's personnel record!" Ira announced triumphantly.

"Keep it down, will you!"

"Sorry."

"Who is he?"

"Marine Sergeant Ramón Delgato. Twenty-eight years old, black hair, brown eyes, six feet five, two hundred fifty-five pounds. Jesus, the guy must be a monster! And look at the training he's had in the marines! Special Forces, qualified on dozens of weapons, tons of survival training. He was in Delta Force."

"That's the antiterrorist strike force, isn't it?"

"That's right. Those guys are bad asses. But they're all gung-ho jarheads and grunts. How'd Camden get someone like him to go along with the program? I mean, these Delta guys are trained to kill, but they ain't homicidal maniacs. And this Delgato is Spanish. Says here he was born in Puerto Rico. Why would he go around killing his own kind?"

David grabbed a few pages off the save pile. "Wait. I was just reading about how they pulled that off. Seems Camden offered Delgato a position the poor bastard couldn't refuse. Sold him on the idea that working for Charlie Camden would be the same as working for the government, only at four times the money."

"So what happened?"

"They conditioned him."

"Drugs?"

"Drugs, sensory deprivation, hypnotism, electric shock therapy, visual and auditory sublims, the entire bag of mind-altering tricks. Then they gave him a new personal history. The guy now believes he was sexually abused throughout his childhood by foster parents. His real parents were supposedly murdered by an uncle. Camden's bunch took this nice, healthy, patriotic guy and turned him into a psychotic killing machine.

"The worst part is that they instilled within him a deep-rooted hatred for anyone of Latin blood. It took them six months to get him where they wanted. Seems Delgato can pass for normal most of the time. But say the trigger phrase, 'Carmen Miranda and the Cisco Kid,' and the dude will massacre anyone he sees who looks Spanish."

Ira glanced over at David. "Like you, for instance?"

David absentmindedly ran a finger through his Vandyke. "Remind me to buy some Clairol Summer Blond before we go after him."

"You mean they let this guy run around loose?"

"No, he's under virtual house arrest here at the installation. They had to leave him with enough brain cells to be able to brief him on the layout of his victims' apartments before they take him in."

"Guess they'd have to keep him from going completely around the bend if they wanted to sneak him into their real target population," mused Ira.

"Yes, it's got to be a pretty ticklish balancing act to pull off. They've left Delgato hanging off the cliff of total insanity, tethered by a slim lifeline."

David held up a finger for silence. A moment or so later Ira heard footsteps approaching down the hall. The steps ended short of the door, paused a moment, then receded as the guard returned from his survey of the cul-de-sac. When Ira looked over at David, he was already flipping through another file. Balls. Brass balls. That was what this guy had.

"This isn't the first experiment, Ira. There's a record of one they ran down in Atlanta back in 1982."

Ira's eyes opened wide. "The Atlanta Child Murders!"

"Time frame sure fits. Says here there's an index with the test targets' names and the dates of the murders. That index ought to be somewhere in this mess."

"God, it makes sense. I remember reading how a lot of the cops weren't completely satisfied that the guy they bagged for those killings did them all."

"If we can find that index we'll know for sure."

"But in Atlanta only kids were killed, not whole families."

"I know. According to these papers Shelley decided to step up the terror factor by killing kids, for greater psychological impact. But the experiment didn't work out as well as they'd hoped. Shelley's notes blame its failure to a great extent on the rural-suburban setting. The crimes didn't affect enough people to create real havoc. At the time, poor blacks didn't have the political muscle in Atlanta needed to sway popular opinion. Project Jack lost its funding shortly thereafter for some unspecified reason, and the experiment was shelved until six years ago."

"Guess that's when Camden found a sympathetic ear in the White House," Ira said sadly.

"At least one in the NSC. That guy turned Camden on to some corporate backers who funded the project. But I'd bet there's some federal money involved."

"During the Reagan-Bush years, the guys with the big bucks thought they could get away with anything, didn't they?"

"Including the overthrow of Castro. That was Camden's original target population, the people of Cuba."

Another guard came along; Ira and David stood motionless until he left. Ira's watch said 1:13 A.M. Apparently security made a pass once every half hour. He and his co-conspirator should be gone before the next sweep.

As he tossed another useless file onto the floor, Ira said, "The Cuban project all makes a terrible kind of sense. The revolutionary government of Cuba has been a sore point with more than a half dozen presidents. The idea of a Communist state less than ninety miles from the North American mainland used to drive that Reagan-Bush crowd nuts. They would have given their right nut for the chance to off Fidel."

"Haven't come across anything that links any real biggies to this project directly. Pity."

Ira ran his tongue around his mouth. Boy, he could really use a cigar right about now. "No way to tell how far up this thing goes from anything we'll find here. You try to make a direct link to the ones in the rarefied atmosphere of the upper echelons of power, they start setting up protective layers of plausible deniability. Imagine sending a psychotic killer to another country to murder innocent women and kids. That's genocide. It's the worst kind of terrorism I've ever heard of. And my own government's behind it."

• David's head suddenly whipped around. Ira froze. Vandemark's expression indicated it wasn't another guard he heard coming their way. Levitt unholstered his gun. David picked up the tire iron off the desk, crept to the door, and flipped off the lights.

A moment later Ira heard a lone set of footsteps coming closer. He sat in the dark, listening to their relentless approach. They stopped directly outside the door. Ira heard the doorknob turn and saw the door open a few inches. Light streamed in from the hall. A man was silhouetted in the opening, pushing on the door, looking down at the floor. Something was impeding his progress: the lab coat. When the man leaned over to determine the problem, Vandemark brought the tire iron down on his head. The man hit the floor with a resounding thud. David hauled him into the room, then he looked out into the hall, listened for a moment, and closed the door.

When the lights came back on, Ira got a good look at the intruder. He was a slim, middle-aged man with close-cropped dark hair, wearing a lab smock. He looked stunned, but he was conscious.

Vandemark pulled him to his feet and tossed him into a

chair beside the desk. Ira, his gun trained on the man, said, "Who we got here?"

"His name tag says he's Dr. James Hoover, Shelley's assistant. One of the masterminds behind Project Jack. Nice of him to show up here so we can question and kill him."

"I said no killing!"

David fixed the massive FBI agent with an icy stare. Ira wondered for a moment whether their partnership was about to end in an exchange of silenced gunfire. He cursed himself for not having made sure there was live ammo in the gun Vandemark had given him.

David shrugged, ending the standoff, and abruptly began stuffing the pertinent documents into his knapsack. "Time to go. Someone might come looking for Hoover. We'll take him with us. When he comes around, he shouldn't be too hard to control."

Coming around was exactly what Dr. James Hoover was doing. His wits were collecting themselves. Ira stepped in closer to cover him. He could see the man's eyes focus. An expression of shock and horror spread across his features when he discerned Ira's towering form before him. Then he saw the gun. In a weak and quavering voice, the visibly trembling man croaked, "Who are you?"

"None of your business, Doc. So keep your mouth shut and you might survive the night. Do we understand each other?" said Ira unpleasantly. It was best to keep Hoover scared, easier to manage. Getting out of the installation was going to be tough enough without anything extra to worry about, like Hoover finding some balls along the way and kicking up a fuss.

Hoover nodded. "I don't want to die. I'll do whatever you ask."

David finished loading up the knapsack, stuffing in as many of the unread files as he could manage along with the essential ones. The knapsack's contents should be sufficient to blow the lid off Camden's nasty plot.

Vandemark turned, giving the doctor his first clear look. Hoover's expression jumped several notches up the sheer terror scale. "You! But you're supposed to be at the apartment!"

Instantly realizing the import of the doctor's words, David grabbed the man by the lapels, making physical contact, and delved deep into the frightened man's thoughts.

Then David grabbed the tire iron off the desk and brought it down again on the scientist's head. No small tap this time. Vandemark hit him with what looked to be lethal force. Hoover jerked, stiffened, and collapsed in the chair. His eyes remained open, but his pupils rolled back into his head. Blood trickled down his face from the split in his scalp.

"What the hell are you trying to do!" Ira roared, turning the gun on David. "I said no killing!"

"If I wanted to kill him, I would have used the gun. I wanted Hoover out of commission for a couple of hours," David said coldly as he put on his knapsack. "We've got no time to mess with him."

Ira checked the unconscious man's neck for a pulse and was relieved to find it strong and steady. Vandemark had had a lot of experience at this sort of thing, apparently.

David was heading for the door. "You coming?" he asked as he stepped out into the hall.

Ira cast a final glance at Dr. Hoover. "Is he going to be all right? I mean, is it okay to leave him?"

"Who gives a shit? Listen, Ira, they've sent the Slasher out tonight. He's heading to the apartment where I've been staying. A really nice woman's life is in danger. If you want to stay and play Florence Nightingale to this lowlife, be my guest." Vandemark disappeared down the hall.

Ira hesitated for a moment, then quickly thumbed the unconscious man's eyes shut and closed the door on his way out.

46

On the far side of the installation Camden, alone in his office, was on the line with McGuire. There was a cellular phone in the tan van outside Angela's apartment. McGuire was giving his boss an update.

"All the lights in the apartment building are out except for the ones in the broad's place, sir. Everyone else retired about an hour ago. They ought to be sleeping soundly."

"Excellent. Go in and get it over with."

McGuire hung up and glanced into the rear of the van. He couldn't see much of Ramón Delgato in the dim light filtering through the fogged windows. Delgato was nothing more than a dark, ominous shape sitting in an only slightly less dense blackness. But this shadow sat quietly, and that was all that mattered to McGuire. As tough as McGuire was, Delgato still gave him the creeps. The brooding giant never said much of anything, but McGuire had seen the aftermath of Delgato's night raids. Messy. Extremely messy. Delgato was a monster, a man-made nightmare. McGuire had the series of coded commands needed to keep this terror in line, but he had no illusions that he'd be able to survive his charge's murderous fury if it was unleashed and directed toward him. McGuire was a trained assassin, one of the best in the business. But this Delgato was inhuman. Nothing short of a howitzer would stop him when he was in the throes of one of his murderous frenzies.

Glad to put some distance between himself and Delgato, McGuire climbed out of the van and walked down the street to where Hanson had the Quinoñes apartment under visual surveillance. Hanson's eyes never moved from the curtained windows when McGuire stepped up behind him and said, "Chief says it's time to party."

Hanson gave a curt nod. "I wish we knew if Vandemark was in there or not. I don't like the idea of hanging around and waiting for him to show up later. Baby always makes such a bloody mess of a place. By the way, how's he behaving?"

"Calm. Let's hope he stays that way."

"You'll be okay as long as you don't forget your command codes."

"Yeah, I guess so. But I'll be glad when this assignment's over."

"Whose turn is it to take Baby in?" asked Hanson.

"Yours. I'll take care of the power."

Hanson gazed quizzically at his partner, trying to decide if he was being bullshitted. He could have sworn he'd taken Baby in last time. But maybe it was the time before. It didn't matter. Hanson wasn't as spooked by Delgato as McGuire was. In fact, he rather liked the brooding giant. Wasn't it Hanson who'd given Delgato the nickname Baby? There was a purity of purpose about Baby that Hanson admired. The brute was a killing machine. Nothing more. Nothing less. Like a shark. The only time Baby came alive was during his bloody sprees. Those scientists had done some job on Delgato. Hanson had to admit he felt sorry for Baby, but he could admire the single-minded drive those shrinks had instilled in the brute. It was like the way Hanson felt about expertly crafted firearms. To him, a finely made weapon was a work of art.

47

Angela Quinoñes was engrossed in a silly 1950s movie. It had taken quite an effort to turn off her worries so she could lose herself in the "drama" of the original *Invaders from Mars*. At least that's what the announcer kept repeating. Angela couldn't imagine anyone wanting to remake a film with this same title, but someone had.

While flipping through the channels, she had happened upon the movie's opening credits. She would have preferred something funny, but there were no comedies to be found, so she had settled on this moldy sci-fi epic, thinking it would probably be campy and good for a few laughs. But she was wrong.

Right from the beginning Angela found herself sucked into the plot. A little boy sees a flying saucer land in a field behind his house in the middle of the night. He wakes his parents, who think he's had a nightmare. Dad checks anyway and finds no flying saucer. Next morning the boy spots his dad in the field. Pop is sucked into a sand pit, to the accompaniment of the weirdest music Angela had ever heard. Shortly afterward Dad reappears at the house, but he's changed. He acts like an emotionless automaton. And he has a scar on the back of his neck. More weird music. The saucer people have done something to him!

From then on, the situation goes downhill. Mom, one of the boy's schoolmates, and some policemen all fall victim to the sand pit and the eerie music. The boy tries to warn folks of the menace, but everyone thinks he's crying wolf. The mysterious aliens are going to take over, and there's nothing the lad can do about it.

Angela found herself completely absorbed by this somewhat surreal thriller. She wasn't even put off when she got a good look at the aliens and they turned out to have zippers running down their rather crusty green backs.

The movie was reaching its climax when the power went out. Angela found herself sitting in the dark with a little white dot glowing in the middle of her dead television screen. Within seconds even that was gone. Angela cursed aloud. Con Edison had struck again. Oh well, electrical outages in the summer were part of the urban experience. But why couldn't they have waited another ten minutes or so? Now Angela wouldn't find out whether the little boy escaped. Would he get his parents back? Would the military save the day? Would the pretty nurse be turned into an alien zombie? Would Angela find a copy of this film down at the video store so she could see how it ended?

Muttering nasty things about the power company under her breath, Angela stumbled to a closet and fumbled around until she located some candles. Then she found some matches and set up a base camp in the living room. After pouring herself another glass of wine she felt fortified enough to begin her candlelight vigil. She wondered how much longer she would have to wait for David to show. Why, of all nights, did Con Ed choose this one to burn out something vital? It was as if the whole world was conspiring to drive her straight up the wall.

Angela told herself to put a halt to that kind of thinking. That train of thought only led to paranoia. The TV stations hadn't plotted to exclude comedies from their late-night schedule just to frustrate her. The power company hadn't timed its breakdown so she wouldn't get to see the end of her silly movie. This was New York City, where these sorts of things happened all the time.

But power outages usually occurred on hot days, she reminded herself as she went to the window, when the demand for electricity was high because everyone was running their air conditioners. Today hadn't been that hot. In fact, the weather had been unseasonably mild.

Angela didn't like what she saw outside. There were lights on in the windows of some apartments across the street. The streetlights were also on. In their icy blue glare Angela saw something that scared the hell out of her.

A man standing on the curb across the street was looking up at Angela's window!

Seconds later a second man joined him, and both of them looked up. Could they see her? No. With her apartment lights out, Angela was sure she was invisible to them. The first man walked up the street to a tan van and got in.

A tan van!

She'd seen it before, but it hadn't registered!

Omigod!

The man opened a sliding door on the side of the van and something crawled out. Or did it step out? Angela couldn't tell. The something was all black. A shadow, with no detail.

Then the first man and the thing walked across the street toward Angela's apartment building. Only then was Angela able to make out that the thing was a man. But he was a monster. He towered over the first man by about a foot. He seemed as wide as he was tall. And he was all in black! Black clothes, black hair, something black smeared across his features. All black. A massive, ominous obsidian shadow.

The two men disappeared below Angela's windowsill. They were heading for the front door of her building. The other man continued staring up at the apartment. Angela's heart was pounding. They were coming for her!

She raced over to the phone to call the police, but the phone was dead.

Those men had cut the line when they killed the power, and now they were coming to kill her!

Why? She didn't know them! She'd never done them any harm! Why would they want to kill her? But Angela had no doubt that that was their intention.

What to do? Break a window and scream for help! No, that wouldn't do her any good, only hasten her death.

Angela opened the door to her apartment and furtively stepped into the hall. She could hear something scraping or scratching five flights below.

Then she heard the familiar creak of the building's front door being opened and carefully closed. Then silence. Total and complete. But Angela knew they were climbing the steps. Coming for her.

She looked down the pitch-black hallway toward the staircase leading to the roof. Should she head that way? No! The men would hear her open the fire door. And once on the roof, there would be no place to run or hide. This apartment house was two stories higher than either of the adjacent buildings. She'd be trapped.

Back to the apartment! She'd be trapped there too, but there were places to hide. It was home territory. She'd have the advantage!

Angela closed the door behind her, heedless of whether they heard. She slipped the police lock into place and pushed a heavy chair against the door. Shoving the sofa against the chair was a lot harder, but she managed, with the help of adrenaline. That would hold them off for a while.

But not forever.

She needed a weapon! Why hadn't she asked David to leave her a gun? But what good would that have done? She didn't know how to use one and might have ended up shooting herself accidentally.

Angela raced to the kitchen. From a drawer she pulled a large butcher knife. Her fingers inspected the sharp, shiny blade. It wasn't much, but it would have to do.

Back in the living room, she blew out the candles. Darkness would help her more than it would her pursuers. The killers couldn't know this place as well as she did. Maybe she had a chance.

Barricades raised, weapon in hand, Angela felt ready. All that was missing was the cavalry. Even an overweight representative of New York's Finest would do. There was only one way to summon this salvation. Scream!

And that was exactly what Angela Quiñones did. She

screamed loud and long. She screamed with every ounce of strength. She screamed with such volume she believed folks in Queens would hear her. She gave it everything she had. Her life depended on someone, anyone, hearing her.

❧

Two floors below, Hanson heard the screams and hissed, "Shit!" He wasn't sure his dark companion heard the noise. Delgato was in his controlled stage, a half-hypnotic trance, responsive only to certain verbal commands, waiting to burst into a murderous rage. He was always transported in this condition.

The sounds of people waking began to issue from the surrounding apartments. Hanson knew the situation was getting out of control. Should he scrub the mission or try to pull it off? Camden would be furious if they blew it.

Hanson shoved Delgato forward, directing him toward the next flight of stairs. He knew McGuire would even now be positioning himself at the front door to contain the building's inhabitants. Without phone service to summon help, a lid might be kept on this mounting bedlam.

When they reached the fourth floor Hanson could hear people stumbling around in their apartments, cursing the power company, asking what the screaming was about. He shoved Delgato along with renewed effort.

And Angela kept right on screaming.

They were almost to the staircase leading to the fifth floor when a man opened his door and asked what was going on. Hanson barked at the interloper, "Police! Get back inside and close the door!"

The man obeyed instantly.

Hanson pulled out his .45 automatic and screwed the silencer onto it. He knew that other tenants would not be so easily handled.

Angela kept screaming.

As Hanson and Delgato were climbing the stairs Angela's next-door neighbor shone a flashlight down on them. "Please hurry!" he pleaded. "It sounds like she's being killed! It sounds like—"

A whispering bullet cut the Good Samaritan off in midsentence. His flashlight bounced on the floor and rolled into a corner, still blazing. The neighbor hit the floor and was still.

And Angela kept screaming.

Hanson hustled Delgato to Angela's door, made him face it. Then he said, "There's a spick bitch in there! Make her stop screaming! She knows you're coming, so don't worry about being quiet! Make it quick! Fast in! Fast out! Carmen Miranda and the Cisco Kid."

It was as if a switch had been thrown. Without the slightest hesitation, Delgato slammed into the door, growling. The portal held, but he immediately crashed into it again and again. The hallway filled with the sound of splintering wood. The door wouldn't hold for more than another few seconds.

The woman stopped screaming.

❧❧❧

Angela raced down the length of her flat, throwing pieces of furniture in her wake. Anything that would slow down the Slasher! Angela reached her bedroom and searched for a place to hide. The closet? No! That door was flimsy. If her front door with its barricades couldn't keep out the Slasher, neither would this weaker one.

Under the bed? No! No room to maneuver.

Behind the bed!

It had a high headboard. That would provide her with protective cover and still give her room to wield the knife. Angela frantically pulled and pushed the bed away from the wall. It banged against her chest of drawers and wedged itself there. Thank God for tiny New York apartments! The Slasher wouldn't be able to move her cover aside.

Clutching her knife, Angela crawled behind the headboard, pulling a nightstand in behind her. The side wall would protect her back.

She heard the front door give way, then the sound of furniture scraping across the floor, being shoved out of the way. He was coming.

∞∞∞∞

Delgato stood by the ruined doorway, panting from exertion. He listened, trying to locate his prey, then pulled a survival knife out of his boot. Its jet-black blade was eight inches long.

She was in here somewhere. He'd find her. The Slasher moved forward on crepe soles, a deadly shadow gliding through the dark.

❧❧❧❧

Angela peered over the top of the headboard, into the darkness, waiting for death.

A bump from out of the pitch-black void. The Slasher had found one of the pieces of furniture she had tossed in his way. Then silence. He was being more careful. But he was still coming.

The butcher knife felt small and ineffectual in her fist. What she needed was an ax.

Something dark moved in the inky blackness. He was at the doorway to the bedroom. Angela silently sank to her knees, every neuron in her body screaming in alarm. Could he hear her panting? She couldn't get her breathing under control, couldn't draw a deep breath. Her lungs burned with the effort.

From her den Angela could hear the Slasher moving around the bedroom. He no longer seemed to be bothering with stealth. The monster was rummaging through the closet, looking for her.

She heard him step toward the bed. She could feel part of his weight press down on the mattress. Then she heard his blade scraping against the floor below the bed. He was sweeping under the bed with it to see if she were there. If she had chosen that refuge . . .

He gave up on that exercise. Silence. He was thinking, wondering where she was. He couldn't see that the bed was pulled away from the wall. Too dark. Maybe he would leave.

And still, the silence.

What was he up to?

More silence . . .

Did he know where she was hiding?

Silence . . .

Then the sound of the Slasher's footsteps heading out of the room! Receding down the hall. Fading.

Silence.

Had he left?

Silence.

Was it safe for her to come out?

Silence.

No. She had to stay hidden until the police arrived.

Silence.

Suddenly something crashed onto the bed, shoving it closer to the wall, pinning her shoulders between the headboard and the wall. The Slasher had returned! He had known where she was all along! He had her!

No!

The Slasher was on the bed. Angela squirmed around to face the headboard and free her shoulders. She pushed herself to her feet, flailing the butcher knife ahead of her as she rose. Angela felt it bite into something solid. The Slasher bellowed in pain.

Something whipped past Angela's face, a mere fraction of an inch away. It had to be the Slasher's knife. She frantically retreated into her burrow, holding the knife above her head.

The Slasher growled and kicked at the headboard, banging it against her. Angela felt her strength fading. Sheer nerve had carried her this far, but it was faltering. She was going to die! The realization hit her like a brick. But she wouldn't cry or whimper. She wouldn't give the Slasher the satisfaction. Nor would she let him kill her without making him pay. He wouldn't escape unscathed this time. She was determined to mark him. With her dying breath she would brand her killer.

Angela sprang to her feet, whipping the butcher knife back and forth, trying to find the shadowy death that was stalking her. The knife sang, but she sliced only dead air. Where was he?

A powerful gloved hand closed around her wrist and squeezed. The pain was overwhelming. Angela heard an involuntary cry of pain escape her lips and felt the butcher knife slip from her grasp. It fell to her feet, a million miles away. And the pain continued.

Angela could feel herself being lifted by the powerful arm that held her prisoner. Her feet left the floor and she helplessly dangled in midair, a lamb ready for the slaughter. It was over.

Somehow, through her pain, Angela managed to open her eyes. Why, she couldn't say. Maybe she wanted one glimpse of her killer. Wanted to see what such a monster looked like.

All she could see in the Stygian gloom were the narrowed whites of the killer's eyes and his teeth bared in a grotesque smile.

Then some type of light flashed out in the hallway and crept weakly into the room. It was enough to silhouette the killer's massive form as it danced along the edge of the black knife about to be plunged into her body.

48

The hole in the floor of the installation's utility room proved to be as good an exit as it was an entrance. Wasting no time, Ira and David crawled out, onto the crossbeam, and into the Hudson River. The river's northern current rapidly carried them away. They swam underwater, coming up for quick gulps of air and immediately submerging again. David hoped no one at the video monitors would spot them. If they did, he and Ira would simply have to shoot their way out. It was a terrible plan, but they had no time to waste on finesse. The Slasher might already be at Angela's.

Chester Pinyon never caught even the slightest glimpse of Ira and David. Flying on amphetamines, his attention span was virtually nil. He was spending more time blathering about what a great artist he was going to be than he was watching the monitors.

Reaching the pier, Ira and David climbed up and raced to the government car waiting on the street. Ira stopped long enough to grab his clothes. The keys to the car were in his pants' pocket.

When Ira caught up with him, David was standing by

the driver-side door, demanding the keys. He wanted to drive, and Ira didn't argue with him. He flipped David the keys as he headed for the other side of the vehicle. Ira thoroughly regretted this decision.

Vandemark tore through the city streets at speeds ranging from fifty to seventy miles per hour. Stoplights and signs flashed by unheeded. More than once David clipped passing cars that weren't quick enough to get out of the way. For the first time tonight Ira was really scared. Breaking into Camden's installation had been a piece of cake compared to this. Ira felt certain that any second he'd find himself scattered all over a New York City street in pieces too small to identify.

Before he knew it they were at Twenty-seventh Street and screeching to a stop. Somehow their insane dash across town had not attracted the attention of a single police cruiser. There's never a cop around when you need one, thought Ira ironically.

As they leaped out of the car, Ira heard David saying something about the top-floor apartment of the building he was pointing at. It occurred to him that his companion had been talking the whole time they'd been speeding over here. But Ira, his mind having been occupied with thoughts of mortality, couldn't remember a word Vandemark had said.

He heard David yell, "God dammit!"

Ira could see that he was looking at a tan van parked across the street. Vandemark pulled his gun and started moving toward it. Ira finally remembered the van's significance and pulled out his own gun. He was watching Vandemark, looking into the van, when the bullet hit him.

It caught him high in the back. Felt like someone had hit him with a sledge hammer. The impact spun Ira around. He caught a glimpse of a man standing on an apartment-building stoop, holding a silenced gun in his hand. Then Ira saw David fire his gun. Little flashes of light spit out of the silencer. The man on the stoop fell to the sidewalk just as Ira himself hit the hard asphalt.

Holy shit! I've been shot! He could see David running toward him, slowing, then running past him. The son of a bitch is going to leave me here to die!

Ira heard breaking glass behind him. Probably that bastard Vandemark kicking in the door to the apartment building.

As Ira lay bleeding in the middle of the road, he pictured how this would look in tomorrow's paper. He could already see the large headlines: FBI AGENT FOUND DEAD IN STREET, WEARING A WET SUIT!

❦

A quick glance at Ira told David that the man was in bad shape, but Angela's peril was more immediate. The Slasher was probably up in her apartment right now. Would he reach her in time?

The front door was locked, so he kicked in the glass, trusting the wet suit to protect him. Inside, he found the hallways filled with confused and frightened people. Flashlight beams danced amid the throng, coming to rest on David. People wanted to know what was going on. What had happened to their electricity? And what was that screaming about?

Screaming!

David grabbed the first man he came upon and ordered him to call the police. "There's a man outside who's been shot! He needs an ambulance!"

"But the phones aren't working!"

"There's a pay phone down on the corner! Use it!"

"But the policeman at the door said we should stay inside!"

David jammed his gun into the man's face. "Do it or I'll blow your fucking head off!" This got the man moving.

A nearby woman who had heard the exchange stepped out of the darkness. "I'm a nurse. You say someone's been shot?"

"Yeah, out in the middle of the street! See what you can do for him!" Then David was gone, racing up the stairs, pushing past blind, frightened, babbling people.

The climb to the top floor seemed to take forever. But as he started up the last flight, he spotted a light at the top of the stairs. It seemed to be coming from the floor, like a flashlight on its side.

Then he caught it: the slightest sensation on the edge of his awareness. But it was enough to make him duck. And that saved his life.

The bullet hit the wall above his head. David's telepathic powers had barely registered the gunman's presence in time. He allowed himself to roll back down half the flight of steps. On his bumpy trip, he caught the muzzle flash of the gunman's second shot. David straightened and ended his roll, slamming his knees against the unyielding wooden steps. He ignored the pain, took aim, and fired.

He was answered by another shot from the unseen gunman. The slug ripped into the step Vandemark was crouched on. David zeroed in on the flash and fired again. A shape pitched over the railing and crashed on the steps above David. He stepped out of the way and let Hanson's dead body roll past him.

Then David heard a crashing sound in Angela's apartment. He took the steps three at a time. On the landing he spotted the flashlight and grabbed it without stopping. He could hear a wailing and hissing noise coming from the apartment. He knew it was Angela. Then someone cried out in pain. That wasn't Angela. The Slasher!

David dived through the ruined apartment door, the flashlight illuminating the way. From the far end of the apartment, he could hear struggling. Shining the flashlight down the hall, he could see a corner of Angela's bed bouncing around. They were in there! Hang on Angela! I'm coming!

He ran about three steps before tripping over a bric-a-brac shelf that Angela had knocked over. But he was on his feet again immediately.

David leaped into the bedroom, his gun at the ready. The flashlight beam lit up the entire tiny room. Caught in the center of the beam was Ramón Delgato, squinting over his shoulder into the light. He held Angela in the air with one hand. His other hand was pulling a bloody knife out of her still body.

David quickly pumped two bullets into Ramón Delgato's back.

49

The two bullets in his back didn't faze Delgato. He dropped Angela behind the headboard and launched himself at David with incredible speed. But Vandemark got off two more shots before the massive ebony giant slammed into him. One bullet caught the Slasher in the shoulder but didn't slow him down; the second shot missed completely.

David twisted aside in an attempt to avoid Delgato's blade, but it cut a red-hot gouge along his ribs. The next thing David knew, he and the giant were scrambling around on the floor. David's breath was knocked out of him, but he tried to bring the gun up and blow Delgato's brains out. He was only halfway there when the giant grabbed his wrist and twisted it. The 9 mm fell from David's grasp. Through a dull scarlet haze he saw Delgato's knife streaking toward his neck. He twisted out from under the madman's great weight, and the blade dug itself into the floor.

David slammed the flashlight against the side of Delgato's head. This only made the behemoth blink angrily. He yanked his knife out of the floor and raised it high to

strike again. David dropped the flashlight and grabbed
Delgato's weapon-wielding arm with both hands. He
managed to divert the bloody knife by shifting his weight
at the last moment, throwing Delgato on his side.

David yanked the killer's arm toward him and bit into
it savagely. This elicited a bellow of anger and agony and
caused the Slasher to drop his weapon. It also got David
hauled to his feet by his hair. The next thing he knew he
was flying across the room. The journey ended when he
landed against the closet door, shattering it. His back
took the brunt of the crash, but he had to give his head a
shake to make the stars go away. Doing this made him realize there was something in his mouth. David spit it out.

The glowing beam of the flashlight gave David his first
clear look at Ramón Delgato. He was even larger than
David had expected. Add fifteen pounds to those personnel-
file vital statistics.

Delgato's clothes, hair, and face were completely black.
Probably greasepaint on his skin. The only spots of color
in this ebony nightmare were a bright scarlet blaze on his
shoulder and the blood dripping between the fingers of
the gloved hand grasping his right forearm.

As Delgato was reaching for his knife, Vandemark exploded out of the closet and kicked the killer in the face.
Delgato went backward ass over heels. David dropped to
his knees and grabbed the knife.

He was only halfway to his feet when Delgato lashed
out with his foot and clipped him on the shoulder. David
crashed into the doorjamb, the knife spinning wildly out
of his hand into the darkness of the hallway. Instantly re-
gaining his balance, he spun toward Delgato, who was
trying to stand up. He brought his closed fist down on the

bridge of the monster's nose with everything he had and was rewarded with a satisfying crack.

He had no illusions about having stopped Delgato. What he needed was a weapon, but his gun was nowhere to be seen. It had bounced under the bed. What else in the room could be used to kill a man?

David caught a quick glimpse of Delgato springing off the floor. He dodged the attack, diving deeper into the room. There was an overturned lamp on the night table that was wedged behind the headboard. David grabbed the light, turned, and slammed it into the charging Delgato's face. The lamp shattered on impact, cutting David's hand as much as Delgato's face. Vandemark followed with a kick to the killer's groin and a left hook to the stomach. The killer merely staggered back a few steps.

Horrified, it dawned on David that he hadn't been using his special gifts so far during the battle. That would have to change. He had to keep out of Delgato's reach. If that giant got his hands on David, he'd tear him apart. Use your brain, he warned himself. If you panic, you'll never leave this room alive!

Contact. But David was forced to pull back from the Stygian maelstrom that was Delgato's mind. He had to keep that deranged intellect at arm's length lest it overwhelm him. A light brush would have to be enough.

He felt Delgato preparing to charge. David had plenty of time to roll onto the bed, out of the juggernaut's path. Ramón smashed into the wall, cracking the plaster. David lashed out, landing a foot solidly on Delgato's jaw, then sprang to his feet and drop-kicked the Slasher into the closet.

Neither combatant landed all that gracefully, but it was

David who got to his feet first. He grabbed a chair and hurled it into the darkened closet. The sound of wood meeting flesh and the accompanying cry of pain were music to his ears.

But there was no more loose furniture in this room, so David sprinted out of the room, hoping to find a weapon in the kitchen. He knew where Angela kept her knives. One of them would look nice sticking out of Delgato's neck.

David's special powers were not able to detect the dangers of overturned furniture. Again his foot caught on an unseen something. He slammed into the wall and crashed to the floor. He was groggily trying to get to his feet when Delgato landed on him like a toppling brick wall.

Even with the wind knocked out of him, David struggled to free himself before the massive killer could get a firm grip. His flailing elbow found the giant's jaw, and David felt the impact clear up to his shoulder. Too bad it hadn't bothered Delgato. The madman grabbed David's shoulder and flipped him onto his back. David saw the descending fist plummeting toward his face; but there was no time to react. The world exploded in pain.

Somehow he remained conscious. His fists lashed out at the giant straddling him, but the blows had lost their power. They thudded against Delgato's jaw unnoticed. David could see the killer grin maliciously as he grabbed David's hands and pinned them under his knees. Vandemark was helpless, trapped beneath his assailant's enormous bulk.

Delgato began to rain a steady torrent of steel hard-fists on David's unprotected face, taking his time about it, making it hurt, none of the blows hard enough to put

David out. Delgato wanted him to feel it coming. Wanted him awake and aware of the approaching end.

David clung to the silky thread of consciousness. Somehow through the veil of pain, he saw Delgato's open hands come toward his face, slip under his chin, and grasp his throat. The powerful hands began to slowly apply pressure. They tightened around his neck, cutting off any chance of a breath. David squirmed, trying to free his own hands, but the effort was hopeless.

He was beaten. The ruthless murderer of four families, twenty-four people, and the woman he loved was claiming him also. He could feel the cartilage in his neck beginning to bow. It would crack soon, and that would be the end of him. With his windpipe closed off permanently, he'd be dead in less than a minute.

Delgato squeezed harder . . .

The world began to fade into an infinite blackness.

Then Delgato's hands slipped away from David's throat.

David's body spasmed, gasping for the welcome oxygen.

He was aware that Delgato was twitching on top of him. David couldn't think why, but at least it let him free his hands.

Delgato suddenly pitched onto his side, his eyes glazed and unseeing. He crashed face first onto the floor, ending up beside David. Angela followed the dead giant as he fell, continuing to stab him in the back with the bloody butcher knife.

50

It took David several seconds to find the energy to get to his knees and stop Angela from chopping Delgato into little pieces. She was striking in a blind frenzy, spitting out a low-volume torrent of Spanish and English curses. David recognized the glint of satisfaction in her eyes. She had even less strength left than he did, so he gently removed the bloody knife from her trembling fingers and led her back to the bedroom.

The flashlight revealed that, though Angela's sole wound was deep, Delgato's knife had not hit any vital organs. He had struck high above the lung, mostly cutting into muscle. Angela would end up with a terrific scar, but alive. By the time David had fetched a towel from the bathroom to use as a compress, Angela, half in shock, was pouring out her story.

"I came to . . . There was all this noise . . . and my shoulder hurt so. Then my hand touched the butcher knife. Everything came back to me. I stood up. I could see . . . what he was doing to you. I got out from behind the bed . . . don't remember how . . . Then I was stabbing him. I couldn't stop myself."

Angela stared into the darkness past the bedroom door. "He . . . he's dead, isn't he?"

"Couldn't be deader. You saved my life, doll. And given half a chance I'll show you my appreciation. Hate to repay you, for now, by running out on you like this," David said in a gravelly voice he could barely recognize as his own. His neck and throat hurt like hell.

It took a few moments for David's words to sink in. "What do you mean? Where are you going?" There was a frantic tone in her voice.

"It's not over yet. The guy you killed was only a part of it. His boss is still out there. I've got to go after him. I'm sorry."

Flashlight beams were probing through the apartment's front door now. They came to a stop in the hallway outside the bedroom. A thin voice squeaked, "Jesus!" David could see the lights playing on Delgato's mutilated body.

"In here!" David called. "It's okay! It's all over. I've got a woman here who needs medical attention."

The beams of light cautiously approached, zeroed in on David and Angela, and were lowered enough to allow David to see the two men behind them. One carried a baseball bat, the other a fireplace poker. "What happened here?" the taller of the two men asked.

David helped Angela stand up and headed her toward the two new arrivals. "Save the questions until the police arrive, fellas. One of you get this lady to a hospital. Either of you see how my partner is downstairs?"

Both men shook their heads, confusion on their faces. David turned back to Angela. "You know these guys? Will you be all right with them?"

Angela nodded.

"Then I've got to go. I'll see you at the hospital later on."

"Will you?"

"I promise."

David stepped past the two men and headed for the door. On his way down the steps, he wondered if he'd be able to keep that promise.

∽∽∾∾

Back in the apartment, the two men helped Angela toward the door. The shorter man with the poker asked, "Do you think we should have let that guy go like that?"

His companion answered, "You got a look at him. Did you want to try and stop him?"

∽∽∾∾

When David reached the street, he found the nurse and a couple of other men kneeling beside Ira. They had removed the top of his wet suit and bound a makeshift compress to his wound. Ira was lying on his side, a blanket folded under his head, another covering him.

David tossed the flashlight into the gutter and walked over. The nurse saw him coming and said, "I think your friend will be all right, if we ever get an ambulance here to take him to the hospital. What's going on in there?"

The night air was filled with the wails of approaching police and ambulance sirens. "Doesn't sound like you'll have long to wait."

"David?" Ira's voice was weak, shaky. David stepped around so Levitt could see him.

"How you feeling, Ira?"

"*Farchadat.*"

"Anything I can do for you?"

"Yeah. Don't let Camden get away."

"You got it."

David turned and walked briskly down the block toward Third Avenue. A number of people who watched him go wondered if they should let this strange-looking man in the wet suit stroll off. But no one seemed interested in stopping him. Why should they? That was the kind of work the police were paid to do. It wasn't their fault there were no cops around.

∽∾∽∾∽

• David rushed into the garage, headed for the upper level where his van was parked, but slowed as he passed the empty attendant's station and caught a glimpse of his reflection in the booth's glass. He was not a pretty sight. His entire face was swollen, bruised, scraped, and bloody. The right eye was puffed up, but his nose had suffered the worst damage. It pointed in an unfamiliar direction and was numb to the touch. David hoped it would stay numb until after he had finished dealing with Camden.

When he reached the upper level, one of the parking attendants spotted him. The man didn't say a word. His eyes followed this bloodied apparition as it headed for the dark van parked in the corner slot.

David pulled a magnetized hide-a-key box out from its place of concealment on the van's frame. Without a word, he climbed into his vehicle, started it up, and drove out of the parking structure. He couldn't resist smiling and waving good-bye to the parking attendant as he passed.

He stopped eight blocks from Camden's installation. It wasn't easy getting out of the wet suit, covered as he was with contusions, but somehow he managed. Every inch of him hurt. It was easier slipping into the loose-fitting dungarees, work shirt, and sneakers. Over the shirt went a bulletproof vest. Then came the weapons: a sawed-off pump-action shotgun, three 9 mm automatic pistols with silencers, and two knives, one a butterfly, the other a throwing blade. He completed his ensemble with a crumpled raincoat, a baseball cap, and a five-gallon can of gasoline.

With the van locked and the alarm set, Vandemark headed down the street toward Camden's warehouse. It was fortunate there were few people on the street at this time of night, because the look in David's eyes would have horrified anyone he had run across.

He wasn't pulling any punches this time. They'd tried to kill Angela. Camden had tried to snuff out the flame of the woman who had brought him back to life.

David had truly believed he and Angela could ride into the sunset after this affair with Camden was over. He had imagined that he could waltz off and eventually lead a normal life. Pipe dream. Now the blinders were off. Even if he managed to take Camden down, this wouldn't be over.

Camden was merely one part of a corrupt system, a network of powerful men without conscience. They backed people like themselves, like Camden. And they knew how to protect themselves. If Camden took a fall, they would move to safeguard their own positions. Anyone who might link them to Project Jack would be eliminated. That included him. And that included Angela if they suspected she might know anything about what David had been up to.

Angela would never survive a war between David and Camden's mysterious backers, David knew that if he survived the night there would be no way to avoid such a confrontation. Which meant that if he lived, it would have to be without Angela. No happy ending. No retirement in a beautiful vine-covered cottage. No dreams fulfilled. All gone, blown away by the cold winds of harsh reality.

There was no more time for recriminations. David was nearly at the door of the warehouse. He'd been striding down the street like a man with a purpose, a man with a destination in mind, somewhere past Camden's installation. He hoped that impression had come across to whoever was manning the video cameras tonight.

∞∞∞∞

Chester Pinyon hadn't noticed David's approach on the monitors. He was still aboard the amphetamine express, talking his fool head off. Braddock had spotted David on one of the screens but written him off as just another nobody heading home after a night out. Looked like he'd run out of gas. The poor slob was going to have one hell of a time finding a service station open in this neighborhood.

But Braddock changed his mind when David didn't pass by the warehouse's main entrance, as expected. Without warning, the guy in the baseball cap threw open the front door and disappeared from view. Braddock called out, "Hey! You know that guy?"

Chester answered, "What guy?"

51

Fred Scully, an unshaven blimp of a man, thought he'd seen everything there was to see come through the doorway he was assigned to guard. In the two years he'd worked for Charles Camden some real weirdos had stepped through that front door—winos, bums, prostitutes, hustlers, druggies, and plain old poor dumb stiffs who'd lost their way. It usually wasn't too hard to get rid of them. Most of them couldn't leave fast enough when old Fred went to work on them. Women, he'd slobber over and paw at. Men, he'd bully and shove out the door. If they got tough, Fred was more than happy to get tough right back. His 280 pound body was not all fat. He'd busted more than his fair share of heads in his time. And he'd done worse.

Fred still remembered that city building inspector. What a moron. The damn fool came in waving his credentials, claiming the owner of this warehouse didn't have the proper occupancy permits. Fred had tried to cool the idiot down by offering him a payoff, which had always worked on other building inspectors. But this dude got himself all worked up and threatened to have Fred arrested for trying to bribe a public official. Said he was going to the mayor's office with this one, demanded to see the building's owner.

So Fred did the only thing he could do. He went over to the file cabinet, pulled out his Uzi, and cut the silly little prick in two. Fred had been dying to see what that machine pistol could do to a body. It'd been everything he'd expected and more.

Of course, Mr. Camden was a mite upset with him. Kept saying the situation could have been handled more diplomatically. But he didn't fire Fred, and Camden's boys got rid of the stiff real professional-like. Fred figured they planted the peckerhead somewhere out in Jersey. Served him right. Camden made Fred straighten up the entrance foyer. He had to plaster over the bullet holes and repaint the dump. But then the place looked too good, so Camden had Fred smear dirt all over the joint again. It was one crazy place to work at, all right. On a job like this you saw everything sooner or later.

That belief was driven home with the impact of a pile driver when Fred saw the guy with the gas can come through the door. One look told Fred he was big trouble. The dude's face looked like someone had pounded it with a meat mallet. And then there were his eyes. Fred had never seen such eyes.

Scully didn't waste time trying to talk to this walking nightmare. He launched himself toward the file cabinet. He needed the Uzi for this one, no doubt about it! His hand was closing around the machine pistol's stock when a single bullet blew out the back of his head. He was dead before he hit the floor. A second bullet shattered the video camera hanging from the ceiling.

⚭⚭

Satisfied that the guard behind the wire mesh partition and the computer-linked ID camera were no longer a threat, David Vandemark set down his can of gasoline and turned toward the door he'd come through. He shot off the padlock that secured the gate to the late Fred Scully's domain. David picked up a chair and wedged it under the bar handle of the front door. It was a solid metal fire door. Jammed shut like that, nothing short of a battering ram would open it.

After retrieving his gas can, David stepped over to the door leading to the heart of the complex and slammed it open with one kick. He immediately fired three bullets into the full-length mirror he found on the other side of the door. A man crashed through the mirror and landed at David's feet. Two of his shots had hit home. David ripped the Uzi machine pistol out of the dead man's hand and stuffed it into one of his raincoat's oversized pockets. He was sure it would be as useful as the time spent picking Dr. Shelley's mind about the installation's security arrangements. This little foray of his wasn't going to be any breeze.

He jogged down the deserted corridor. There were a few doors along this hall, but David sensed no one behind them. This hallway led into another. Vandemark knew Camden's office was down the hall to his left. But the pleasure of making the man's acquaintance would have to wait.

A set of double doors at the other end of the corridor led to the installation's barracks. That was where most of Camden's hired goons would be at this hour, relaxing, waiting for a call to arms. David took off his belt and wrapped it around the two door knobs. He knew this measure wouldn't hold off a determined group of well-trained men for long, so he poured the contents of his fuel can over the twin portals and tossed in a lit match. That end of the hall disappeared in an explosive conflagration. David knew there was another exit from the building through the barracks, but at least Camden's gunmen wouldn't be able to get back into the building through the front door and sneak up behind him. Not without announcing their intention with dynamite first.

Smoke detectors set off a deafening din. Ignoring it, David raced down the hall to Camden's office. He kicked opened the outer door. Three men were there, getting up out of their seats to see what all the noise was about. As soon as they saw David they went for their guns. One of them managed to clear his holster before David cut him and his buddies down with a 9 mm fusillade.

Hearing voices in the hallway, David left the office and found two men stepping out of doorways he'd passed on his way. Both men had their backs turned to him. They were looking at the raging fire at the other end of the hall. One of them turned, saw David, and went for the gun under his sport coat. David pumped two slugs into both men.

Stepping back into Camden's reception room, David tossed the empty pistol on a sofa. From his coat pocket he extracted the Uzi, checked to see the safety was off, and kicked open the doors to Camden's inner office. He sprayed the darkened room with machine-gun fire. David heard someone cry out in mortal agony over the ripping sound of the Uzi discharging its deadly load.

Being careful not to allow any survivor a clear shot at him, David flipped the light switch by the door. There were no survivors. A beefy man lay dead on a sofa off to one side of the room, a shotgun on the floor next to the couch. Probably a guard catching a nap in the boss's office.

David knew the other body lying sprawled across the large desk wasn't Camden's. Not with that red hair. The man was much too young to be his quarry. He wore a blood-spattered lab coat and clutched some papers in his stiffening hands.

Damn! Somehow he had missed Camden! Now what?

As he stepped out of the office, David pulled the sawed-off shotgun out from under his raincoat. No need for stealth. Anyone who didn't know he was here was either deaf or dead.

If Camden was in the barracks for some reason, he was lost to David. There'd be no way to find him. But David's end of the hallway turned to the right. This hall led to the science labs, security offices, a loading bay, the utility room, and the stairway to the second floor. If Camden was down this way, there was still a chance to bag him.

But Camden wouldn't be alone. He'd have security guards with him, and they would soon be joined by any of his gunmen with enough sense to head for the loading dock once they found they couldn't get in through the front door.

A man came around the corner, brandishing a shotgun. David fired his first, slamming the gunman against the wall. The dead man left a crimson streak as he slid to the floor.

The hall was filling with blinding smoke. Nowhere to

go but forward. David raced around the corner and crashed into two more of Camden's security men. All three of them tumbled to the floor, a tangle of flailing arms and legs. David managed to slam a foot into the face of one of them. Then David rolled, came up on his knees, and fired two quick rounds in their general direction. The second shotgun blast caught the conscious guard as he was trying to get to his feet. David didn't waste a shell on his partner, as the man wasn't going anywhere.

The air was a little less dense down this way. So when the door to the monitor room opened, David didn't immediately blast away at it. Braddock stuck his head through the doorway. Vandemark clubbed it back into the room.

He hadn't connected hard enough to put the burly security guard out, so he kicked the door fully open and trained his shotgun on the prone Braddock, whose gun lay on the floor beside him. He'd dropped it when he got that nasty purpling bruise on his forehead. Braddock shook his head and stared in disbelief at David. Vandemark smiled back. "Braddock, isn't it? Hi. Remember me?"

Braddock answered by lunging for his gun. The shotgun blast took most of his head off.

"Please! Don't shoot! I'm going to be a great artist!" pleaded Chester Pinyon, cowering in a corner. "I haven't done anything wrong! I only watch the monitors!"

David could see from Pinyon's muddled thoughts that he was telling the truth. But he covered him with the shotgun anyway. David motioned for Chester to head for the door. Chester obeyed, babbling incessantly about his innocence and what a great destiny awaited him in the art world. When they reached the hall, David said, "You're not going to have any kind of destiny if you don't get out of here. The place is burning."

David stopped Chester from running toward the front of the building. "Wrong way. That's where the fire is." Chester nodded frantically, turned, and ran toward the back of the warehouse, thanking David over and over again for sparing him. He promised David that he wouldn't be sorry. Chester Pinyon would someday be a household name.

Not if one of Camden's trigger-happy goons cuts you down, thinking you're me, thought David as he watched Chester disappear into the thickening smoke. Never one to pass up a golden opportunity, David decided to follow twenty or so paces behind this very obliging goat.

But first he drew the second of his handguns out of his pocket. The shotgun was clumsy in tight quarters.

⤞⤜

Chester got halfway down the hall before it occurred to him that his troubles might not be over. There was a gun battle going on. That horribly bruised man had killed Braddock! Someone had invaded the installation! But who? Communists? The man back at the monitor room looked neither Chinese nor Russian. He had dark skin and jet-black hair. The man could be a Latino, a Jew or maybe an Arab. *Arab!* They were Arab terrorists! That had to be it. It made perfect sense.

This was awful! Chester could get killed! The battered man had let him go. But his comrades might not be so understanding.

Worse yet, one of the security guards might accidentally shoot *him*, Chester Pinyon, possibly the greatest painter to ever walk the face of the earth! They might mistake him for one of the invaders and kill him before they got a good look. It would be easy enough to do in this dense smoke. And that would be a terrible tragedy!

There was only one way to avoid this dreadful misfortune. Chester began to wave his arms wildly as he continued to run, screaming, "Don't shoot! This is Chester Pinyon! I'm not a terrorist! Don't shoot! My death would be a terrible loss to the art world!"

Joe Bates reached out through an open doorway and grabbed Chester by his shirtfront. It nearly stopped the young man's heart. "Please! Please! Don't hurt me! I'm an artist!"

"Shut up!" Bates growled, his face, ugly and twisted with anger, only inches from Chester's. "What the fuck's going on out there?"

"Arab terrorists! They're everywhere! Killing everyone! Braddock's dead!" Chester whined miserably.

"What the bloody hell are you talking about? What Arabs? Are you trying to—" Joe Bates's face exploded, showering Chester with blood, bone, tissue, and gray matter. His lifeless hand released its iron grip on Chester's shirt, and the young artist who wanted to be Jackson Pollock resumed his mad dash down the smoky hall, screaming, "The Arabs are coming! The Arabs are coming! Run for your lives! Run!"

David pocketed the 9 mm as he approached Joe Bates's still and bloody form. He relieved the dead man of his Uzi and headed off again in Chester's wake. That boy was working out just fine. A regular Paul Revere. Arabs indeed.

⋙⋘

The security guards in the loading dock heard Chester coming long before he stumbled out of the smoky hallway into their line of fire. Many of them felt like peppering his hide with lead by way of greeting. His screaming had been getting on their nerves. But Luke Styles, the head of security, had ordered them to hold their fire. They had no idea what was going on inside the installation. Most of the men with Styles had come from the barracks. All they knew was that the warehouse was on fire and that gunfire was being exchanged. Styles wanted intelligence before he committed himself to any action. The screamer might at least provide some information.

Chester was hustled away from the hall doorway and drawn behind the hastily prepared ramparts Styles had his men throw together out of crates, boxes, and barrels. The frantic artist kept blathering nonstop about Arab gunmen as he was dragged along. "Where's Mr. Camden?" Chester pleaded. "You've got to tell him! Shiite terrorists have stormed the installation!"

Styles slapped Chester roughly across the face. "What's going on in there?" he demanded.

"You gotta tell Mr. Camden that the Arabs are here!" Chester repeated, only temporarily shaken by the blow.

"You'll tell *me* what's happening, you little twit! Got It? Camden's still somewhere inside the installation. *I'm* in charge here! So talk!"

Chester started babbling incoherently about dead gorillas, Arabs, fires, Russians, exploding heads, and Jackson Pollock. Styles was getting ready to slap Chester again when a shotgun blast hit the security chief.

Four more shotgun rounds from the hallway followed; David saw no point in wasting time on 9 mm finesse. Everyone ducked for cover except Chester, who broke free once more and raced for the open door. As he charged through the loading dock out into the clean night air, he managed to thank, individually, all the celestial powers for his salvation.

The loading dock was ablaze with automatic gunfire. The barrage ripped into crates and cartons, sending splinters and Styrofoam peanuts flying in every direction. Two men were wounded. The majority of the security force hit the floor, but a few returned the fire and it wasn't long before the rest of them joined in, emptying their guns, slapping in new mags, firing, reloading, firing. The leaderless men lacked the sense to stop shooting long enough to see if they were getting any return fire. So the loading dock filled with a deafening crescendo.

∽∾∿∾∽

As soon as he'd emptied the second Uzi, David dived into the hallway that ran parallel to the loading bay, and not a moment too soon. The defenders' return fire ripped through the doorway and walls. David left the empty shotgun and Uzi behind and crawled along on his belly as plaster and splinters rained down all around him. About a hundred feet or so down the hall he felt safe enough to get up on his feet and run for the staircase leading to the second floor. That had to be where Camden was hiding. Fate had given him another crack at the man.

David felt the teeniest twinge of remorse about shooting Luke Styles after the man had been so obliging as to inform him that Camden was still trapped in the burning building. But Styles had bragged about being in charge, so David had had no choice in the matter. He needed confusion to help keep Camden's cutthroats off his back. He hoped it would be a while before another of their number chose to take up the reins of leadership.

The air inside the warehouse was nearly unbreathable. The open loading-dock door was providing the raging inferno with all the oxygen it would ever need. Temperatures throughout the warehouse were rising rapidly. As David climbed the steps, he wondered if he had to worry about going after Camden. The fire had already broken through to the second floor. Perhaps Camden was dead?

A bullet caught David in the chest, and he pitched backward down the stairs.

❦

Charles Camden had been looking for Dr. Hoover when all hell broke loose. He wanted to talk to Hoover about any problems the scientist might foresee in moving Project Jack out of the country after the New York tests were completed. Normally he would have called the doctor down to his office, but the tripling of the security force had overcrowded the installation's barracks. The off-duty guards were being allowed to sack out on any sofa they could find. Because of that, Camden had decided it would be easier consulting with Dr. Hoover in his own office, which had no sofa.

He hadn't found Dr. Hoover. So Camden decided to see if perhaps the missing scientist was in the late Dr. Shelley's office. He was about to turn the office's doorknob when the fire alarm sounded. What the devil?

On his way down the stairs, Camden heard the roar of the Uzi. He froze in his tracks. Vandemark! It had to be David Vandemark!

The blasts of a shotgun followed. Camden pulled the Springfield Omega out from beneath the well-tailored lapels of his Armani suit and checked the load. Eight rounds in the mag. One in the pipe.

More gunfire. Getting closer. Camden wondered what to do. A .45 caliber round from his gun would stop any man. But from the sounds reaching him he could tell that much heavier firepower was being used downstairs. He remembered that FBI agent saying that David Vandemark had tracked down twenty serial killers and executed them. Camden wished he'd been more thorough in reading Vandemark's FBI file. A superficial reading of the reports had convinced him that Ira Levitt was an incompetent agent trying to cover his failings by exaggerating the skills of the criminal he'd failed to apprehend over seven long years.

Now Camden wasn't so sure.

The crazy bastard had invaded Camden's fortress and torched it, if the thickening clouds of smoke were to be believed. Camden decided to exercise the better part of valor and let his men handle the intruder. He raced back up the stairs and through the upper floor, heading for the front steps, away from Vandemark.

The front stairs led to the installation's barracks. Camden was horrified to find hungry flames dancing their way up that stairwell. Damnation! He'd have to use the rear stairs after all. Maybe he could reach the loading dock and get out of the warehouse that way. His men would regroup there if the barracks were on fire. Camden couldn't stay here. The entire second floor was rapidly being consumed by the geyser of flame pouring from the stairwell. Why had he chosen such a rickety death trap for his headquarters? Camden was choking on the smoke. He ran blindly through it. The air cleared somewhat as he reached the rear stairs.

Then he heard more gunfire. It sounded dreadfully close by. Not far from the stairs. A shotgun at first, answered by an Uzi. Then dozens of guns being fired at once. It sounded like World War III. Camden gazed down into the stairwell, racking his brain for a way out of this fix. And that was how, through burning eyes, he happened to spot a man racing up the steps. He knew instantly that it had to be Vandemark.

He quickly drew a bead on the runner, following him up the steps. As David rounded the landing and started up the second flight, Camden fired. He caught Vandemark square in the chest. The psychopath pitched backward onto the landing and lay still as stone on the floor. What else could he do? thought Camden with satisfaction. No one got up after taking a .45 in the ticker.

But David Vandemark did. He bounced up without warning, filling the air with 9 mm fire. Camden dived away from the stairwell's handrail. "The son of a bitch ain't human!"

❧❧❧❧

David Vandemark was decidedly human and well aware of the limits of that condition. The bulletproof vest had stopped the slug, but not before it had cracked a couple of ribs. The wheezing he heard when he breathed was no longer caused by the thick smoke alone. David was rapidly reaching the end of his rope. If he was to get Camden it had to be now, before he collapsed. It took nearly everything he had to continue climbing the steps.

David sensed Camden around a corner, waiting to ambush him as soon as he set foot on the second floor. Big deal, Vandemark. You don't need to be a telepath to figure out that move. David fished his third and last gun out from beneath the raincoat. The second 9 mm was empty.

Smoke was getting thicker, and the heat was draining him of strength. David pitched the empty pistol at Camden.

When the gun hit the wall, next to Charles Camden's head, he ducked back behind the protective cover of the corner. It was an involuntary response that left him cursing his reflexes as he stepped forward to regain a bead on his nemesis.

But David Vandemark had made it to the top of the stairs. He fired as soon as Camden showed himself. The bullet caught Charles Camden in the upper right arm. His beautiful nickel-plated Springfield Omega slipped from between numb fingers.

Camden turned and raced down the burning hallway, hoping to find a way to escape. What hope did he have against a man bullets didn't stop? Better to take his chances with the fire.

Fire danced along the walls. Camden could feel the smoke-filled air sear his lungs. He ran through flames. The back of his suit was beginning to smolder. Blisters were rising on his face from the heat. His hair felt like it was on fire. And then suddenly he could run no farther.

A rolling wall of heat and flame pushed its way down the hallway, forcing him back. Back toward David Vandemark. Camden turned, knowing what he would see. Yes, there he was! Vandemark!

Vandemark, the killer of killers. Camden's judge, jury, and executioner. Justice. Death. Never in his wildest imaginings had he thought his end would come like this. He'd hoped death would be quick and painless. He never dreamed he'd come to the end of the road feeling so scared and helpless.

David Vandemark was serenely walking along the flaming corridor, seemingly oblivious to his own singed hair and smoldering clothing. The gun in his hand hung loose at his side. But his eyes—they smoldered. They blazed with hatred. And they burned deep into Charles Camden. This vision was unmistakable. Here walked the Reaper. Something wet ran down Camden's leg barely noticed. Death. There was no escaping it. So Charles Camden decided the only sane thing to do was get it over with. He began to stumble toward the wild-eyed demon that would end all his fear and pain. "Do it, you bastard!" he screamed. "Get it over with!"

David Vandemark leveled the gun at his target. Charles Camden tensed for the bullet that would sever him from his life. Then all at once there was a loud cracking, ripping, grating sound. Camden felt the installation shudder under his feet.

Vandemark seemed to sense what was about to happen a fraction of a second before the floor he was standing on collapsed. But he was too late. His shot went high, missing Charles Camden by a good foot. Camden stared in dumb amazement as his tormentor vanished from view, leaving behind only a sagging, splintered hole in the floor though which flames licked up. He had been granted a reprieve!

But it would be wasted completely if he didn't get out of here quickly. His right arm hanging useless at his side, Charles Camden stumbled up the corridor, coughing and hacking. He slid along the wall to avoid following Vandemark to his fiery doom. Thick smoke billowed from the hole in the floor. The fire was much worse downstairs. But it didn't matter much because Charles Camden would be out of this inferno within a few more seconds. All he had to do was reach the stairwell and get to the loading bay, where he would be safe.

But then something grabbed his leg.

It was Vandemark.

The lunatic had managed to get a handhold on the burning flooring, had avoided dropping into a flaming death on the first floor. He was pulling himself out of that smoking pit now hand over hand, climbing up Camden's leg as Camden watched, transfixed in his terror.

Vandemark was a horrible sight to behold. His hair was scorched, frizzed off in every direction. The skin on his hands and face was smoke-blackened, cracked, and bleeding. But his eyes still blazed with an infinite fury as he pulled himself up . . . up . . . up. . . .

Camden's strength deserted him. He fell against the burning wall and slid to the floor. Ash and fiery cinders showered down on him unnoticed. The only thing in the whole universe he was aware of was the monstrous apparition scaling his leg. It couldn't be human! It couldn't!

From somewhere deep inside his desperation, Charles Camden found the strength to raise his other leg and slam his foot into the monster's face. He couldn't believe it when Vandemark loosened his grip on his leg and the devil slid back into the smoky hell pit from which it had sprung.

Camden stumbled to his feet, unable to accept his good fortune. He fell down part of a flight of steps because he kept looking over his shoulder as he went, expecting at any moment to see Vandemark spring out of the flames at him. Then, before he knew it, he was in the loading bay and could hear somebody screaming, "Hold your fire! It's the chief!"

Hands grabbed him and helped him through the bay, out through its doors, into the cool, clean, life-giving air. His body shook, and he nearly collapsed as he was seized by an uncontrollable coughing fit. But his men kept him on his feet, moving him steadily away from the heat. Camden heard someone going on about Arab terrorists, but he paid no attention to it. Walking, even with help, required all his concentration. His head was swimming as he was helped into a car.

The clean air rapidly cleared Camden's muddled thoughts. Someone was saying something about getting him to a hospital, but he waved them away. Charles Camden, leaning wearily against the car door, turned around to look at his installation, the home of Project Jack.

The entire building was a gigantic ball of flame. Police and fire trucks were on the scene. Popping flashes amid the gathering crowd proclaimed the media's presence, but the reporters were keeping their distance from the burning structure. The sound of gunfire had kept even the cops and the firefighters at bay until they figured out what was going on. By that time it was too late for them to do much. Within the hour the warehouse would be nothing but a smoldering ruin. Everything was gone. Everything. Six years of Charles Camden's life had gone up in smoke. Project Jack. Camden was certain Dr. Hoover was inside that inferno. That meant no rebirth of the project was possible. The alchemist's oven was useless without the alchemist. The fire had taken it all.

But Charles Camden didn't care.

Because that same fire had also claimed David Vandemark.

PART FOUR

Legacy

I am ready to meet my Maker, but whether my Maker is prepared for the great ordeal of meeting me is another matter.

—Winston Churchill

52

Angela was rushed into the emergency room. She wanted to lie down in a nice soft bed. And she wanted to see David.

The knife wound was probed, cleaned, stitched, and bandaged, as were several other abrasions. Angela was wheeled off to a semiprivate room and given the bed of her dreams. A smiling nurse appeared presently with pills for Angela to take. To her surprise and indignation, this nurse was informed that her medicines were unneeded and unwanted. Angela was determined to wait until David's arrival before slipping off to drugged oblivion. The persistent nurse assured her the pills were only a mild sedative. Angela wanted no part of them. She was getting her spirit back.

So a doctor was summoned. He insisted that Angela needed the medication. She'd suffered a nasty injury. Her body required time to rest and recuperate. If Angela didn't take the pills he would prescribe an injection. Angela didn't think the doctor could legally do that, but she gave in anyway. Her renewed spirit could carry her only so far. Within minutes she felt a numbing calm descend.

As she lay in her hospital bed, pleasantly floating, the doctor returned with two policemen. They were arguing. The doctor kept repeating that Miss Quiñones was in no condition to answer their questions. The policemen were adamant. They were investigating a murder, they said, as if that overrode any other consideration. Angela faded before the debate was settled. She knew that her leaving the realm of the conscious would put an end to the discussion.

Angela's dreams were filled with haunting images. The pictures overlapped and superimposed themselves on one another, making it impossible for her to read anything into them or see them clearly. And there were the sounds—a turbulent bedlam of screams, crashes, scraping noises, and explosions that reached a maddening volume and then merged into a high-pitched screech, which in turn metamorphosed into a dreadful wail of anguish coming from the blackened lips of Ramón Delgato.

Angela Quiñones bolted upright in bed, instantly awake and trembling. But the madman wasn't there. No one was. She was alone in the semi-private room, the other bed empty. Morning light streamed between the half-closed window blinds. Angela was in the hospital. The Slasher was dead. She was safe. And David would soon come to her. She would lie back and rest a bit before he arrived. Angela wanted to be fully awake when she saw David. They had so much to talk about. So much . . .

She fell back into a peaceful, dreamless sleep. Nothing disturbed this rest until the voice came to her. It seemed to be calling to her from a great distance. She had to strain to hear the words, but she recognized the voice. It was David.

He sounded desperate. He was warning her about something, but she didn't understand what. David kept repeating that Angela was in danger. She should answer no questions, pretend she didn't know anything. Her life depended on this.

Angela strained to awaken. She had to find out what David was talking about. There were so many questions. It was hard to escape the gossamer chains of sleep that bound her, but she refused to give up the struggle. A nameless fear fueled her efforts. She strove for consciousness. And finally gained it.

But Angela was alone. The room was empty.

She hadn't awakened quickly enough. David was gone.

Angela called his name softly. The only answer was the door of her room slowly opening.

David?

No. It was a smiling nurse. The woman stepped into the room and said, "So you finally decided to wake up. You slept for nearly twelve hours. How are you feeling?"

Angela said nothing. She kept remembering David's voice. It sounded so frightened, so anxious. She remembered his words.

The nurse stepped over to the bed and took Angela's pulse. "Are you feeling any pain?"

Angela looked blankly into the nurse's eyes and asked with all the sincerity she could muster, "How did I get here?"

"You don't remember?"

"Not a thing."

53

Vida Johnson was torn reluctantly from her sleep by the phone. Her wristwatch said 4:18 A.M. A glance at the window confirmed it was not yet light outside. Lieutenant Nyberg, the head of the Slasher task force, was on the line. "Are you awake?" he asked.

"I . . . I am now. What's up?"

"Your partner's been shot. Get down to Bellevue."

Vida hung up. She was dressed and out on the street, hailing a cab in less than five minutes. Nyberg and a score of other police officers were waiting for her at the hospital.

The only good news was that doctors had wheeled Ira out of surgery with the pronouncement that his prognosis was excellent. The 9 mm slug had lodged in his shoulder blade. No vital organs had been touched. A month from now Ira would be on his feet and back at work. Well, she thought, that prediction remained to be seen.

The NYPD had many questions that needed answering—promptly—and Vida was hustled off to another room. Why had Ira Levitt, FBI agent, been running around Manhattan in a wet suit, for chrissake? What had he been up to? The man who had been with Ira at the time of the shooting fit the description of someone tentatively identified as David Vandemark. But this Vandemark had been killed later on in a warehouse fire on the West Side. Shots had been fired during that incident. The city investigators were trying to piece together what had gone down. Did Vida know whether Ira's investigation had led him to that warehouse for any reason? She answered truthfully that for the past few days Ira had been working on something on his own. He hadn't wanted to talk about it. Could she see him? The answer was no. He was heavily sedated, in recovery.

Then some FBI agents from the New York office showed up. Vida didn't know them. The same questions were repeated, and Vida answered them again. But the agents wanted to know if she'd ever been to the warehouse that had burned down tonight. No, she had no idea even where it was located. Had she ever heard of Charles Camden? Vida recalled reading his name somewhere in the news. Something to do with the White House, wasn't it? What did he have to do with Ira's shooting? The agents nimbly ducked the question.

Her performance was flawless.

Cover your butt, she told herself. And try to cover Ira's oversized rear as best you can.

The agents wanted to know whether she and Ira had uncovered any connection between Vandemark and Arab terrorists. Arabs? Why, no.

The interview continued along this line for fifteen minutes or so. From their questions, Vida slowly inferred what had happened earlier that evening. It didn't look good. Ira was going to have to talk a blue streak to get out of this one.

Vida was telling her fellow agents for about the fifth time that she had never heard Ira say anything that could be considered sympathetic to the Palestinian cause. For chrissake, Ira was Jewish! That was when the tall man in the extremely well-tailored navy suit stepped out of the elevator. Alarms went off in Vida's head. The man spoke to Lieutenant Nyberg. They were too far away for Vida to catch any of their conversation, but something about the man held Vida's interest.

In the back of her mind Vida frantically juggled ethical dilemmas. How much did she owe Ira? How much of herself was she expected to sacrifice for her family? It sure looked to Vida as if someone was going to get short-changed.

The newcomer called the FBI agents away and left her sitting alone for a moment. Then the tall man came over and repeated the questions the others had asked her. His low-key, controlled tone disturbed Vida greatly. This guy exuded power. Though Vida knew nothing about this nameless stranger, she was willing to bet a week's pay that he was a Washington big shot. CIA maybe?

When he finished his questioning, the tall man dismissed the FBI agents and the New York police. He suggested that Vida go back to her hotel and get some rest, but she found the courage to say she wanted to stay for a while to see how Ira was doing. The man told her that the doctors had assured him Ira wouldn't regain consciousness until sometime in the afternoon. Vida said she wanted to stay anyway. Ira was her partner. The man nod-

ded his understanding, said good-bye, and stepped into
the elevator.

Vida waited sixty seconds, then made a mad dash for
the fire stairs. She caught up with Lieutenant Nyberg in
the parking lot. "You've got to assign a guard to Ira!" she
told him. "He might suffer a fatal accident if he's not
watched carefully."

"What are you talking about? Vandemark and the
Slasher are dead. Who'd want to hurt Levitt?"

"Maybe someone in a dark blue suit."

"Do you know something you haven't told me?"

"No. But I think a lot of other people are holding back.
Why would a federal hotshot show up at a shooting involving a low-level FBI agent?"

"Federal hotshot? Is that what that guy is?"

"It's written all over him. He ordered you to hold off
your investigation into this matter, didn't he?"

"Through his FBI stooges, yeah. What's going on
here?"

"I think Ira stumbled onto something big here. It may
be cover-up time. Ira's a cop, sir, just like you and me.
Don't you think we owe him some protection?"

Nyberg fell silent, lost in his own thoughts. At last he
said, "I'll send two men over right away. You keep an eye
on Levitt until they get here, okay?"

"Thanks." Vida nodded and headed back into the hospital. On her way up in the elevator she pulled her service revolver from her purse and checked its load. She
kept remembering something Ira had said to her on the
day of their split. The words kept playing tag with each
other in her mind.

"I'm tired of playing at dealing justice," he said. "It's

time I took a chance on the real thing." She'd asked what that meant, and he'd replied, "Maybe you'll figure it out someday, Vida."

Was today the day?

Vida's mother and brothers popped into her thoughts. But Ira's smiling face also crossed her mind's eye. Damn you, Ira, she thought. I don't deserve this. It's too much to lay on me. I've got responsibilities, people depending on me.

But Vida knew she would have a lifetime of sleepless nights ahead of her if she turned her back on Ira. He deserved better.

Damn it to bloody hell! Sometimes the only choice was no choice at all.

∾∾∾∾

The police guards arrived at the hospital within the hour. Their orders were directly from Lieutenant Nyberg. No one was to relieve them without their hearing from Nyberg in person. This took a great weight off Vida's mind. Ira would be safe, for now at least.

Vida didn't think her staying would do any good. She would check in on Ira later this afternoon. Some quiet time was called for. But on her way to breakfast she passed a newsstand. Every front-page headline was either about the fire or the shooting of an FBI agent. Vida picked up a copy of each paper and retired to a nearby coffee shop to study them.

The official story was that the warehouse had held Social Security records. That was why no one could explain the late-night raid and the torching. The terrorists apparently thought they had stumbled onto something much bigger. At least twenty people had died in the blaze. The media were calling it the worst terrorist attack since the Oklahoma City bombing. It still hadn't been determined how many of the victims were Arab terrorists. Some of the bodies could have been washed away in the tide after the warehouse collapsed into the river.

There was a sidebar about the wanted American fugitive, David Vandemark, who had led the Arab attack. Vandemark had been sought in connection with twenty murders in eleven states. There was no mention that the alleged victims had all been serial killers.

Arab terrorists? Where the hell did they come from? Vida wondered. Were they some kind of joke? The press didn't seem to think so, but the papers did report rumors that a radical Shiite Muslim organization was claiming responsibility for the raid.

A spokesman for the White House was quoted as saying they feared this might be the beginning of massive terrorist action within the United States in response to the recent arrest of certain notorious Middle East terrorists. And he reminded the press corps that the State Department had been warning of such a possibility for months. He promised that if proof was found as to who was responsible for this outrage, the appropriate steps would be taken. The spokesman refused to elaborate on what those steps might be.

Vida left her breakfast half eaten and retired to her hotel room. The morning news on the tube was filled with the two related stories. There was speculation that the wounded FBI agent was somehow connected with the terrorists. What was he doing in a wet suit on East

Twenty-seventh Street? Why hadn't he reported to his superiors lately? Vida nearly kicked the television screen in. Report to what superiors? No one in Washington wanted to know what she and Ira were up to!

She was about to shut off the tube when Chester Pinyon came on one of the early-morning shows. He was the hero of the hour. Supposedly the young man had risked his life to warn his fellow warehouse workers about the Arab attack and had pulled several people from the burning building. Vida remembered seeing Chester's face in a photo in one of the papers. He and some other men were helping an unidentified man away from the fire. Chester's had been the only face turned toward the camera.

But this Chester Pinyon was not only a brave young man; he was an artist as well. And he had been kind enough to bring along some of his paintings for the viewers' enjoyment. They were awful. And Pinyon sounded like a real ass, besides. Vida flipped off the set.

My God, Ira, she thought. What have you gotten yourself into?

54

Two detectives came to the hospital to question Angela that afternoon, but she couldn't tell them much. Yes, the detectives had talked to the doctor. They understood she was suffering from trauma-induced amnesia, couldn't remember a thing that had happened to her over the past week, but they wanted to talk with her anyway if she felt up to it.

Fifteen minutes later the two detectives were sold on Angela's amnesia act. She suggested it might stir her memories if they told her a little about this David Vandemark, the man they were asking about. The two policemen decided it couldn't hurt. "After all, Vandemark's dead," one of them said. "For all intents and purposes that case is closed."

Angela forced herself to conceal her horror at this news.

"Yeah, Vandemark killed twenty people," the cop told her. Angela sensed the detectives knew more about these killings than they were saying, but she didn't pursue it.

The policemen told her how lucky she was. "Why lucky?" she asked.

"Well, Vandemark didn't kill you. Most folks who met this guy ended up dead." The detectives told how Vandemark had died leading a terrorist commando raid on a government warehouse. The lunatic had joined up with a bunch of religious fanatics against his own kind. He and his pals had bought it in the ensuing fire.

But what connection did Vandemark have with the Latino Family Murders? she wanted to know. One of the nurses had told her it was the Slasher who had tried to kill her. The detectives had to admit they were still trying to figure that one out. This case was pretty confusing.

As the detectives were getting ready to go, Angela enquired if Vandemark's body had been recovered. Was there any chance that he was still alive?

"No way!" one of the detectives assured her. "The coroner's office hasn't positively identified all the dead yet. That job will probably take well into next week. But there's no doubt whatsoever that Vandemark's dead. You got absolutely nothing to worry about on that count."

Angela cried for an hour after they left.

But she'd heard David's voice last night! It couldn't have been a dream! His words echoed clearly in her mind. There had to be a mistake somewhere.

They hadn't found his body. She felt certain that David had somehow gotten out of that burning warehouse. He wasn't dead. Angela couldn't allow herself to consider that possibility. Without him there'd be no reason to go on. If there was no body maybe there had been no death. David *had* spoken to her.

As the day dragged on and no David Vandemark appeared at her door, Angela began to be tormented by doubt.

That evening when the nurse brought her sedatives, Angela hid them under her tongue. When the nurse left, she spit the pills into the bathroom sink and rinsed them down the drain.

55

Ira regained consciousness around one o'clock that afternoon but almost instantly drifted off to sleep. Vida prayed her partner was playing possum. The tall mystery man in blue and two FBI agents were circling the waiting room like buzzards. They wanted to question Levitt at the earliest possible opportunity. The doctors were going along with the program. This head vulture clearly had the clout to get whatever he wanted.

Please, Ira, she pleaded silently, please be faking this little snooze of yours. Come up with a good story, and make sure you have it straight before they set these scavengers loose on you.

❧❧❧

Ira Levitt opened his eyes at three in the afternoon and demanded to see someone from his office and his partner, Agent Vida Johnson. There was some discussion regarding Vida's presence in the room, but Lieutenant Nyberg had arrived by then and he saw no reason why she should be excluded. He demanded to be present during the interview as well. New York was his jurisdiction, his bailiwick. The mystery man relented, with the proviso that if it looked as if Levitt's story was moving into classified matters, both Johnson and Nyberg were to leave immediately. He was firm about this and refused to elaborate.

Ira didn't look so good, but Vida was overjoyed to see him alive. He told his fairy tale in a slightly slurred voice, stopping often to rest.

Ira had been looking for a snitch who hung out around Times Square. He never found this guy, but he got the surprise of his life when he ran into David Vandemark, the felon he'd been hunting for seven years. Vandemark was talking to some guy. Imagine, seven years of tracking this Vandemark across the whole country and Ira runs smack into him on a Times Square street corner. What were the chances? But by the time Levitt made it through the crowd, Vandemark had disappeared among the passersby. No trace of him. But the guy Vandemark had been talking to was still there, buying cigarettes at a newsstand. So Ira decided to follow him, hoping this character might lead him to Vandemark.

Vida interrupted Ira's story to ask if the man he was following was an Arab.

Ira caught the look in Vida's eye and said, "He might have been. I never got real close to him, but he could have been an Arab or maybe an Indian. From India."

The man in the blue suit told her to withhold her comments; *he* was conducting this interview.

Ira related that he'd followed this second man over to the West Side docks, watched him enter a van waiting there and emerge a few minutes later in a wet suit. The guy then went to the end of the pier and jumped into the river. From a hidden vantage point, Ira watched this character swim around under the warehouse for about half an hour. Then he returned, climbed up onto the pier, got back into the van, and drove off. Unable to find a cab, Ira lost the guy.

Ira was curious about what this character had been up to under the warehouse. So the next day Ira got his car and bought a wet suit of his own, but the lead went nowhere.

The man in the blue suit asked if anyone had given Ira grief about swimming around under the warehouse. "Why, no," replied Levitt. "Didn't see anyone. It's pretty deserted around that part of town."

The Washington big shot was obviously not satisfied with the answers he was getting. Despite his visible displeasure, he said, "Please continue, Agent Levitt."

Levitt was happy to oblige.

He was getting back to the car after his dip, he said, when Vandemark and the other guy showed up. Ira's gun was in the backseat with his clothes, and he was still wearing the wet suit. So he scrunched down in the front seat, out of sight of Vandemark and his pal.

The two of them talked for a bit, then got back into their van and drove off. Ira followed them over to East Twenty-seventh Street. There was no time to call for backup. Vandemark and the guy had gotten out of the van and were heading for an apartment building. Ira was afraid he'd lose them. He grabbed his gun and went after them on foot. The next thing he knew, he was lying in the street with a bullet in his back. He had never seen it coming. That was all he remembered.

Blue suit and his flunkies had Ira repeat his story twice.

But the burly FBI agent stuck to his version. You say witnesses claim I spoke with Vandemark after the shooting? That's news to me. I must have been delirious. Wonder what we said.

By the time they called it quits, Vida could see that Ira's interrogators had bought nine-tenths of the fabrication. They left Vida in the room, saying they'd be back to wrap up the details.

"How'd I do?" asked Ira when they were alone at last.

Vida smiled. "You're a good liar, Ira."

"Thanks. You can't imagine what it means to me, hearing you say that." Ira glanced around the room. "Think it's safe to talk? Bugs, I mean."

"I think so. Nyberg's had a couple of guards on the door ever since you came out of surgery. This was the first time the suit was allowed in here."

"Okay, then. Tell me about what's been going on. What did I miss while I was napping?"

Vida told him everything she'd learned, deduced, and theorized since the previous night. She could see Ira's sadness when she told him of David Vandemark's death.

"I'm sorry, Ira."

"Yeah . . . but at least he saved his girlfriend."

"She's in this hospital, you know. One floor up. She has traumatic memory loss, they say. Can't remember a thing about Vandemark."

Ira shook his head sadly. "Maybe that's for the best. It'll keep her from getting tangled up in this mess with Camden."

"Speaking of Charles Camden, his name hasn't popped up in any of the papers or on TV. When those men questioned me, his name came up once and was never mentioned again. This is smelling more and more like a cover-up to me."

"I'm afraid your pretty little nose is right on the money, Vida."

"You and Vandemark never found any proof of what Camden was up to?"

"Tons. But it all disappeared with Vandemark," Ira told her.

"Then Camden walks?"

"Looks that way. Guess the good guys don't win this time, but at least we closed down Project Jack. That's something, anyway."

"Project Jack?" Vida asked.

"Better you don't know anything about it."

"If you say so. Is this the end, Ira?"

"It will be if we play our cards right. But I'd feel more secure with a gun nearby."

Vida slipped her 9 mm under Ira's pillow. Then she fluffed it for him. Levitt smiled. "Thanks, partner. You came through for me when I needed you. I appreciate it."

Vida could feel tears welling up in her eyes. But before they fell, Ira said, "Now get out of here. I want to get some rest. I'm a sick old man."

"That's right. I forgot. I'll see you tomorrow."

"Great! Bring some magazines and a deck of cards. I'll teach you how to play poker."

Heading for the door, Vida turned and said, "I might teach *you* a thing or two about the game, Mr. Levitt."

෴

As soon as he was alone, Ira pulled Vida's gun out from under the pillow and checked it. He wished he had his own, of course, but this would have to do. At least Vida would be out of it. He slipped the gun under the sheet, beside his thigh. They'd be coming soon. Men like Camden didn't leave loose ends dangling, and Ira didn't believe for a moment that his story had gotten him off the hook. Camden couldn't take the chance that Ira might know more than he was telling. The fairy tale had bought him, at best, another day or two of life. But Vida's gun would allow Ira to take one or two of Camden's errand boys with him.

56

For Ira the night passed without incident. The same could not be said for Angela. So she slept late.

More police and FBI officials came to ask them questions, to which Ira and Angela gave the appropriate answers. The mystery man in the blue suit did not make an encore appearance. There were bigger fish that needed frying elsewhere. Vida began to hope everything would work out after all. Ira knew better, but he kept this to himself.

The nurses who visited Angela's room found her distant and moody, but her vital signs were strong and her wound seemed to be healing. The entire staff was aware that Angela Quinoñes in room 317 had been through a lot. It was only natural for her to feel out of sorts. She deserved a chance to retreat from the harsh realities of the world for a while. They would keep an eye on her. If she needed a sympathetic ear, one would be made available.

Besides, the staff had their hands full keeping a small army of reporters from getting to her room. Miss Quinoñes had become an overnight media sensation. The press wanted to know all about the woman who had been living with the late David Vandemark, the deranged serial murderer. But Angela wanted nothing to do with them, so the nurses dutifully kept the journalistic hounds at bay.

Vida returned at nightfall to keep Ira company with a few games of chance. At least that was her stated purpose. She had sensed his tension during the day and thought perhaps he wasn't clueing her in on everything. It might be a good idea to stay close to him for the next few days. That was all the time she had left in New York City.

She had been reassigned to a new case, in Las Vegas of all places. She'd be joining a task force investigating organized crime within the casino industry. Ira congratulated her on the billet. It looked as if her sentence in Siberia had been commuted. He breathed a sigh of relief. Vida would be out of town when they came for him. At least he wouldn't have to worry about her.

And so they gambled for toothpicks, chatted, and passed the early evening in each other's company. No telling when they'd see each other again. But they were parting friends. That was good. They were both surprised at how much that meant to them. It remained unspoken. Firm resolutions were made to stay in touch, but both wondered if they'd be able to keep those promises.

Ira faded around nine o'clock, right in the middle of a hand of hearts. Vida sat for a few moments listening to his ragged snoring. The big man put on a good show, but it was obvious his injuries had taken a lot more out of Ira than he was willing to let on. Well, have yourself some sweet dreams, you ol' walrus, she thought. You've earned them.

There was a knock on the door. Vida's right hand disappeared into her purse. "Yes?"

One of the police guards stuck his head in the door. "He up for an unexpected visitor?"

"Who is it?" Vida asked, protective of her sleeping companion.

"Says her name's Angela Quinoñes."

Quinoñes? What did she want? Vida shrugged. "Search her and let her in."

"Got nothing on her except a bunch of papers in this bag," the policeman informed Vida a moment later as he ushered Angela in. Surprised to see that the Quinoñes woman was wearing street clothes, Vida waited for the policeman to close the door before she said, "Do the doctors know you're up and about?"

"No, and if you tell them it might mean my life."

Now what did that mean? Vida could discern no answers in the Quinoñes woman's pinched features and intense stare. "Why don't you have a seat and tell me about it."

Lowering herself gingerly into a chair, Angela replied, "I haven't got time for any chitchat. Came by to give you this."

Angela held out an overstuffed backpack. Vida opened it and began leafing through the papers inside. Then she came upon Delgato's personnel record. Her jaw dropped as she stared at Angela. "This what I think it is?"

Angela nodded sadly and said, "Proof of what Project Jack was all about and Camden's connection to it. It's all here in Dr. Shelley's files."

"How did you end up with them?" Vida asked in amazement.

"I snuck out of the hospital last night and got them from David's van." Angela was looking down at her hands, seeming to study them.

"Guess he told you about them after he saved you from the Slasher," said Vida.

"Something like that. David Vandemark was a remarkable man. Much more remarkable than you suspect, Miss Johnson. There was so much I didn't know about him. So much no one will ever know."

Tears began to roll down Angela's face. She pulled herself together, clearly by an act of will, and continued. "He wanted Charles Camden to pay for what he had done. David wanted that more than anything. It cost him his life. I guess it's up to us to finish the job. Do you have any problems with that?"

"Miss Quinoñes, do you know what you just handed me? Either a bull's-eye to paste on my back or a one-way ticket back to the professional gulag. Yeah, I got plenty of problems with that."

"I was supposed to give the papers to Agent Levitt."

One corner of Vida's mouth turned down in a half grimace. "The man ain't up to the burden right now."

"How about you?"

"Don't know. I need to think this through. What're you planning on doing?"

"Disappearing."

Vida thought it was worth a shot. "We can get you into a witness protection program. That way—"

"A *federal* witness protection program? I might as well shoot myself in the head. I don't want anyone in the federal government to know where I am. Listen, you and

Agent Levitt will have your buddies and your guns to protect you. My only armor is going to be anonymity."

"But—"

"This is a nonnegotiable point."

Recognizing a lost cause when she confronted one, Vida merely said, "Good luck, then," and she looked down once more at the papers on her lap.

Angela rose and walked to the door, opened it, and turned back to Vida. "What are you going to do with the file?"

"Maybe the right thing. I really don't know."

"Good luck to you too, then."

Vida looked up in time to see the door close.

Ira continued to snore gently.

❧❧❧❧

Little brothers waiting for a future she was supposed to provide.

Richard Davenport telling her she'd have to sleep with him if she didn't want a lousy quarterly performance reevaluation.

Mom carrying on about responsibility.

Charles Camden, one of the biggest old boys in the old boy network.

Ramón Delgato standing over the bodies of slaughtered Latinos.

That cramped little office in the basement, down the hall from the morgue.

"I'm tired of playing at dealing justice. It's time I took a chance on the real thing."

"What does that mean?"

"Maybe you'll figure it out someday, Vida."

❦

Angela took the elevator down to the lobby and left the hospital. No one noticed.

She started walking to the parking lot on the next block. It was an unbearably long walk. Her strength was rapidly deserting her. Angela needed to lie down, but she knew she would make it. She had to hang tough for a little while longer.

When she reached the van, she discovered that two cars had parked so close there was no way to get in through either of the side doors. No problem. One of the nice things about a van was its back door. She pulled the keys out of her pocket, unlocked the rear doors, and, with an effort, climbed in. A few moments later she backed the van out and drove out of the lot. Angela Quiñones was on her way to a new beginning. A new life.

❦

Vida Johnson stepped out of Ira's hospital room, the backpack slung over her left shoulder. The guard, sitting on a folding chair beside the door, looked up and asked, "Calling it a night?"

"Guess so. Can you do me a favor?"

"What's that?"

"When Ira wakes up, can you tell him I said good-bye? Tell him I'm off to take a chance on the real thing. He'll know what I mean."

"Sure, no problem."

Outside, Vida found the nearest pay phone. Digging around inside her purse, she located her phone book and enough change for the call. Byron Laker answered on the third ring, sounding a bit on the sleepy side.

"Byron, it's Vida."

"Vida! How are you doing?"

"I could use some help. Are you still with the attorney general's office?"

Suddenly fully alert, he answered, "I sure am. What's up?"

"I'm in New York, heading for the shuttle to Washington. I'll meet you at your place for breakfast. Tell you about it then. Don't—I repeat, *don't*—tell anyone I'm coming."

"Are you all right, Vida?"

"I should be if you keep your mouth shut until I get there."

"You've got it."

"You're terrific, Byron. Thanks."

Placing the receiver back on its cradle, Vida thought to herself, Well, that was the first step. They say it's always the hardest one to take.

57

"Holy shit!" Byron Laker finished reading another page from Dr. Shelley's file. "You realize what kind of dynamite you just laid in my lap?"

"Sorry about that, Byron. Couldn't be helped." Vida poured herself a third cup of coffee.

"They'll bury this and both of us, Vida. Charles fucking Camden! Jesus! And a senator and former NSC member! This will never see the light of day."

Vida took the time to savor another sip of coffee before answering the challenge. "They can't stop us this time, Byron. I've already seen to that."

"What do you mean?"

"I got into Washington at midnight. Time enough to get myself some life insurance. I spent the rest of the night waking up close, trusted friends—six of them. Gave each of them a package to keep. Each package contains a copy of that file and a letter of explanation. Each package is sealed, addressed, and stamped. If anything happens to me those friends have been instructed to drop those packages in the mail."

"I don't want to know where those packages will be delivered, but I've got a feeling you're going to tell me anyway."

"Four of them are addressed to the news divisions of ABC, NBC, CBS, and CNN. The last two will go to the *Washington Post* and the *New York Times*."

Rubbing his head as if he felt a headache coming on, Byron Laker said, "That smacks of blackmail, Vida."

"Blackmail, insurance—sometimes the dividing line between such things is extremely slim. Don't you think it's time you got on the phone and woke up your boss? I'm sure he'll find that file awfully interesting reading."

Getting up from the table and heading out of the room, Byron muttered, "Sure, why not. No reason why I should be the only one developing an ulcer this morning."

58

The stretch limousine cruised along I-95 at a good ten miles above the speed limit. The chauffeur wasn't worried about being ticketed for this minor infraction. He knew most traffic cops had the good sense not to pull over a big boat like this. Why waste time writing a ticket that would never be paid? Cops realized people with cars like this were so well connected they were immune to the banal annoyances of everyday life.

The driver eyed his passenger in the rearview mirror. These men had other problems to deal with. The guy in back had plenty on his mind this morning.

Charles Camden sat ramrod straight in the backseat, oblivious to his luxurious surroundings and the passing New Jersey landscape. He wasn't a happy man.

It wasn't his injuries that bothered him, though the cast on his right arm was cumbersome and the arm beneath it did itch like the dickens. He didn't even care that most of his hair had been shaved off, too singed to save. The ointment the specialists had given him for his blistered hands and face was soothing and cool on his skin. A pill, taken once every four hours, eliminated most of the discomfort from the injuries he'd suffered in last night's fiasco. No, his worries weren't physical. The best medical care money could buy had seen to that. But Charles Camden did have problems.

Something was definitely wrong. But the trouble was that Charles Camden didn't know exactly what. He'd only seen the symptoms thus far. The malady itself remained a mystery.

This morning Camden had left New York City feeling on top of the world. But as the day wore on, that world had begun to crumble. He was heading back to Washington. Project Jack was finished. Time to move on to something new. The experiment's failure would not be held against him. A wild card had been thrown into the deck. It was almost an act of God. Could have happened to anyone.

Besides, Camden had left no loose ends that might embarrass anyone of importance. Such tidiness was appreciated by the people Charles Camden associated with. A project might not work out. That was okay as long as you cleaned up your own mess afterward. The ultimate sin was getting caught.

So Camden began his leisurely drive to Washington by making some business calls on the limo's cellular phone. It was time to call in some favors and line up a new venture. He'd been kicking around a number of ideas in his head over the past few months. A couple of them had some definite possibilities. Camden wanted to bounce them off a few people whose opinions he trusted.

But when he called their offices he was greeted by the icy voice of a receptionist who claimed her boss would be out for the rest of the day. The first time this happened, Charles Camden thought nothing of it. The second time, it seemed odd but nothing to get concerned about. When he received the same response on the third call, he began to wonder. On the fourth call he noticed the receptionist's tone didn't cool until she found out who was calling. He then received the message: "Mr. So-and-So won't be in for the rest of the day. Sorry."

Camden went through four more similar exchanges before abandoning the futile exercise. He couldn't believe it. He was Charles Camden. Cabinet members made time to receive his calls. People didn't *duck* him. Charles Camden was a mover and shaker, a bigwig, a doer, a hotshot.

He was in trouble.

But what kind of trouble? What had gone wrong? How could he fix it?

Camden quickly punched in the phone number of his private office in Washington. He recognized the forced joviality in the voice of Marianne Hostetler, his private secretary. Yes, everything was fine at the office, she said. Everything was under control. But something odd had happened. All six of the men Mr. Camden had appointments to see later in the week had called to cancel. Each had a different, equally lame excuse. Though she said nothing, Camden knew Marianne sensed trouble coming. If you work in Washington long enough you get good at reading the handwriting on the wall. Charles Camden hung up, stared unseeingly out the window, and brooded. How had he screwed up?

When the phone rang half an hour later he nearly jumped out of his cast. He let it ring four times before he picked it up. Marianne was on the line. She was frantic. "They came in, handed me some kind of legal paper, and started taking everything," she told him. "There was nothing I could do to stop them!"

Camden slipped into his cool, detached leadership mode. "Settle down, Marianne. Who came in? What did they take?"

"They took everything! Your files! All the papers in your desk! Everything! They said they were federal agents!"

"What kind of federal agents?"

"They didn't say, and I didn't think to ask. I'm sorry, Mr. Camden."

"That's okay, Marianne. I understand. Why don't you close up shop and go home. I'll be in contact with you."

Camden hung up the phone and stared at it fretfully. It was all coming apart. They were coming after him. The wheels of the machine were beginning to grind.

The phone rang again, but it sounded muffled. It stopped ringing before he could pick it up. That was when he noticed that the chauffeur was speaking on a cellular.

Camden pressed the button to lower the glass partition between himself and the driver. The chauffeur was listening, occasionally responding with a curt "Yes" or "I understand." He finally signed off with a "Will do."

After a few minutes of grim silence, Camden asked, "Who was that?"

The driver looked in the rearview mirror and said, "Just the motor pool, sir. They've got another assignment for this boat. Wanted to know what our ETA was."

"Nothing more?"

A pause.

"No, sir."

Charles Camden raised the glass partition, though he knew it would offer little protection when the time came. He was certain he would never reach Washington.

59

SIX MONTHS LATER
WILLOW, NEW YORK

Ira Levitt drove the rented Toyota up the long, winding driveway, directly to the front of the house. He got out and surveyed the property. It had been a long trip.

He'd started off at a Washington, D.C., car-rental agency, coming in unannounced and plopping down cash for the rental. From there he'd driven to New York City, making only two stops along the way—at a McDonald's take-out window and a self-service gas station. He wasn't about to let the rental car out of his sight for a second. No one was going to slip any radio transmitter into it. If they tailed him they'd have to do it the old-fashioned way. No hi-tech monkeyshines.

Ira was sure he'd lost any conventional shadow on the meandering route he'd taken through Manhattan. But just to make certain he had zigzagged around Jersey for a while before heading for the New York State Thruway. When he was satisfied that he wasn't being followed, he headed for Willow and a long-overdue visit.

It was a nice place. A cute little cabin with what looked like a new addition on the side. Someone had been doing some landscaping. New shrubs dotted the property. Two freshly tilled flower beds ran along the front of the house. Cozy. The place looked like the home of a happy couple. Ira hoped it was.

As he stood there, a redheaded woman stepped out from behind the house. She was wearing work gloves and carrying a pair of garden shears. When she spotted Ira, she froze in her tracks. He was sure she recognized him.

After several interminable seconds, the redhead began to walk toward him. As she neared, she said, "Hello, Ira." There was little warmth in the greeting.

"Hello, Angela. You're looking fit. How's the shoulder?"

A redheaded Angela Quinoñes stared evenly at her visitor for several seconds. At last she said, "Fine. It's healed nicely. I go by the name Ali these days."

"I know. I like Angela better. But if you prefer, I'll use Ali."

"Please. How did you find me?"

"Day after you left the hospital, I called a guy I know at the Bureau. He's a whiz with computers and owed me a few favors. I had him flag your medical file at Bellevue. Figured you might want your records. When you tapped into Bellevue's computer my pal was able to trace the line here."

"So this friend of yours also knows where I am?"

"No, he just picked some info out of the data banks for me. He's a full-blown electronics nut. The only periodicals he ever picks up are filled with schematics, not lurid tales of murder and beautiful women. The name Angela Quinoñes didn't mean anything to him. You've got nothing to worry about on that front."

"Then you've known where to find me for quite some time now?" she said quietly.

"That's right."

"Why'd you wait until now to visit?"

"I thought I'd let things settle down a bit before stopping by."

"From what I read between the lines in the newspapers, it doesn't sound like the Slasher scandals are going to settle down for some time yet."

"That's right. The closed-door Senate hearings are slated to begin next month. That'll stir things up again. But I doubt they'll uncover anything new. It looks like Camden's direct contacts are as far up the ladder as they're going to get on this one." Ira motioned toward some nearby lawn chairs and said, "Mind if we have a seat? I have trouble standing around since I got that bullet in the back."

"Oh, I'm sorry. Yes, of course," Angela said as she led the way. When they'd gotten settled she asked rather brusquely, "Any leads on Camden's whereabouts yet?"

Ira shook his head. "No, and I don't think there ever will be. The man is a loose end. I figure he's planted somewhere in the Jersey Pinelands or maybe next to Hoffa in Giant Stadium."

"I hope so," Angela replied with real feeling. A moment later she added, "I read about that senator stepping down."

"Yeah, for reasons of ill health and IRS trouble. Lot of that going around the Hill right now. A certain former NSC member skipped the country last week because of the same problem. That didn't make the papers, though. Thought you'd like to know."

"Will any of them be charged with anything?"

"On the federal level: misappropriation of funds, conspiracy to defraud, perjury, that sort of thing. New York State will probably get into the act later, add a few felony counts to the list."

"No murder charges?"

"No, Washington likes to wash its real dirty laundry in private. The big boys figure ruining the guilty is punishment enough."

"Does that mean they won't do any jail time?"

"Who knows? But one thing they won't get is a presidential pardon. Not this time. Thanks to Vida."

"Good for her. How's she doing?"

"She's been attending a lot of secret congressional and Senate hearings, and she's plugging away at getting her law degree. She's doing okay."

This about exhausted their area of mutual interest, so they drifted into an uncomfortable silence, filled with one unanswered question, Angela watching Ira, Ira glancing around the yard like a prospective buyer. But at last he broke the silence. "Where is he?"

"Right behind you with a gun pointed at your head."

Ira turned cautiously to take a look and immediately recognized David Vandemark, despite the sandy hair and full beard. Ira could faintly see the burn scars David must have picked up in the warehouse fire. The nose was different. Looked as if it had been broken and badly set. But David was smiling. Ira returned the smile and said, "You don't need that cannon, you know. Haven't we already pointed enough guns at each other? I mean, we never ended up using them, so why bother?"

David's grin broadened, and he lowered the gun. He

joined them on a lawn chair and tucked the pistol into his belt. "Where's that partner of yours?"

"Back in Washington. A secret like this should only go so far."

"Thanks, I appreciate that."

"How about a couple of cold brews, guys? Christ, I could really use one myself." Angela turned without waiting for a reply and headed for the house.

The two men kept grinning foolishly, each glad to see the other. David was the first to speak. "Ira, did you ever buy the story of my demise?"

"No, but I'm probably the only one who didn't, David. Or should I call you Vic?"

"Either one. I've spent so much of my life under assumed names I'll answer to just about anything."

"Okay. Well, as I was saying, I knew about that hole in the utility room floor. Never told anyone, though. I heard you fell through from the second story. Is that right?"

"Yeah, I landed only a few steps away from the utility room. Scorched the hell out of myself, but I got out alive."

"Everyone bought the story of your death because they wanted you dead so badly. It made everything much tidier, much easier to accept. The idea of a psychotic killer exposing a government-run one-man death squad made things too complicated. The press would never buy it. Neither would John Q. Public. Why should the big shots be any different? The whole mess being accidentally uncovered during a botched terrorist raid was much easier to swallow."

"No one at the Bureau suspected my demise was maybe a little too convenient?"

"If they did, they kept their mouths shut about it. They were more than glad for the chance to close one of the longest-running active cases they'd ever had."

"What about Camden's crowd?"

"My guess is they feel the same way. If you are alive, they've got no way of finding you. So it's easier, neater for them to file you under *D* for dead."

"Well, I for one am more than happy to continue fostering that misconception. That is, unless you have any objection to my doing so."

Ira shook his head, a wry smile playing around his lips. "None whatsoever. I didn't come up here to drag you back to testify before some damn fool Senate subcommittee. I'm only here to confirm your continued existence, strictly for my own edification."

"What about your duty to the Bureau? Doesn't letting one of the bad guys get away look bad on your record?"

Angela came out with three frosty bottles of Corona and handed Ira his as he announced, "I retire from the Bureau next month. Besides, if they reopened your case, poor Vida would probably be assigned to it. Wasting one career tracking your worthless hide is enough. But what about you, David? What are you up to these days? Still in the game?"

David looked at him and knew it was not an idle question. He decided to let his new wife answer it.

Angela threw an arm around David's shoulders and said, "No way! He's retired. Permanently." Then she quickly glanced at David for confirmation.

"You heard the lady," he said. "All my hunting equipment is stored away in the attic, never to be used again. I traded in my van for a station wagon. What you're looking at, my good fellow, is a man of leisure."

David could feel enormous tension drain from Ira's thoughts. Levitt deserved a break. In a way, the FBI agent had helped end the career of the villainous David Vandemark. There would be no more hunts. No more vigilante kills. Serial killers were once again the purview of the police. And David Vandemark's charred bones lay at the bottom of the Hudson River. There was no one here but Vic Tanner, ham actor. Nothing to worry about from this guy. He might step on your lines, but he wouldn't hurt a fly. Ira Levitt could retire without worrying about any past indiscretions returning to plague him.

The FBI agent sat forward in his chair and raised his glass with renewed enthusiasm. "Retirement. Ah, that word is music to my ears. In fact, I'd go so far as to say it calls for a toast! Here's to retirement, the golden years. May they be many, long, and thoroughly enjoyable. Here's to the good life!"

Three bottles of Corona clinked together.

"Yes, to the good life."

"Hear, hear."

"*L'chaim.*"